Workbook
to accompany
Surgical Technology
Principles & Practice

Fourth Edition

PREPARED BY

CHRISTINA L. BAUMER RN, PhD, MEd, CNOR, CHES
Chair, Division of Continuing Education
Program Director, Surgical Technology
Lancaster General College of Nursing and Health Sciences

NANCY H. WRIGHT, RN, BS
Program Director, Surgical Technology
Virginia College, Birmingham, Alabama

JANET A. MILLIGAN RN, CNOR
Program Manager, Assistant Professor for Surgical Technology
College of Southern Idaho

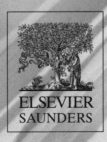

ELSEVIER
SAUNDERS

ELSEVIER
SAUNDERS

11830 Westline Industrial Drive
St. Louis, MO 63146

WORKBOOK TO ACCOMPANY SURGICAL TECHNOLOGY
Fourth Edition
ISBN: 0-7216-0497-8
Copyright © 2005, Elsevier Inc.

Notice

Surgical technology is an ever-changing field. Standard safety precautions must be followed, but as new
research and clinical experience broaden our knowledge, changes in treatment and drug therapy may
become necessary or appropriate. Readers are advised to check the most current product information
provided by the manufacturer of each drug to be administered to verify the recommended dose, the method
and duration of administration, and contraindications. It is the responsibility of the licensed prescriber,
relying on experience and knowledge of the patient, to determine dosages and the best treatment for each
individual patient. Neither the publisher nor the author assumes any liability for any injury and/or damage
to persons or property arising from this publication.

Publisher: Michael S. Ledbetter
Developmental Editor: Katherine V. Judge
Publishing Services Manager: Jeff Patterson
Development & Production: Triple SSS Press Media Development, Inc.

Printed in the United States of America

Last digit is the print number: 9 8 7 6 5 4 3 2 1

Preface to the Student

This workbook is designed to help you apply and master key concepts and skills presented in *Surgical Technology: Principles and Practice, 4th Edition.* Material you've studied in each chapter and in class will make more sense and you'll remember more after completing the variety of exercises included in this workbook.

You'll find exercises specially tailored to help you master objectives in both the theory and practice of surgical technology:

▶ A **key term review** starts each chapter. This includes a comprehensive list of important words in each chapter and tests your knowledge of their definitions.
▶ **Labeling** and **drawing exercises** help you practice the details of anatomy and the skills of surgical technologists.
▶ A variety of questions test your knowledge of concepts in the book, including **matching, true/false,** and **multiple choice** questions.
▶ **Short answer** response questions apply what you've learned to a variety of situations.
▶ **Case studies** help you practice the on-your feet, practical skills of being a surgical technologist. Patient case scenarios take you one step closer to joining the medical community.
▶ **Skill Evaluation checklists** help you monitor your progress and can be used by your instructor to evaluate your competency. These are designed to accompany the skills presented in the textbook.
▶ **Internet Exercises** guide you in finding answers to current, important patient care and health issues facing the medical community today. You'll gain valuable knowledge and hone your skills in finding high quality medical information using the Internet.

Best wishes as you begin your journey to become a surgical technologist.

Contents

v

Chapter 1
The Surgical Technologist

Key Terms

Write the definition for each term.

1. ACS: _____

_____

2. AORN: _____

_____

3. ARC-ST: _____

_____

4. AST: _____

_____

5. Back table: _____

_____

6. CAAHEP: _____

_____

7. Case-cart system: _____

_____

8. Circulator: _____

_____

9. CST: _____

_____

10. CST-CFA: _____

_____

11. Delegation: _____

_____

12. Dependent tasks: _____

_____

13. Flash sterilize: _____

_____

14. Independent tasks: _____

_____

15. LCC-ST: _____

_____

16. Open a case: _____

_____

17. Proprietary school: _____

_____

18. Scrub: _____

_____

19. Sharps: _____

_____

20. Sterile: _____

_____

Short Answers

21. What event is associated with the development of the role of trained surgical personnel?

_____

_____

22. Why did this event require specially trained non-nursing personnel?

_____

_____

23. What were these personnel first called?

_____

_____

24. At about what time did formal schooling of these personnel begin?

_____

_____

25. When was the AST formed?

_____

_____

26. At about what time did the title of these trained personnel change to surgical technologist?

_____

_____

Matching

Match each term with the correct definition.

A. care and empathy

B. manual dexterity

C. honesty

D. organizational skills

E. respect

_____ 27. The ability to coordinate actions and limit unnecessary motion when preparing for a surgical procedure

_____ 28. The ability to be truthful in one's actions and communications

_____ 29. Being polite and courteous to patients, coworkers, surgeons, and others

_____ 30. Demonstrating compassion and a willingness to truly listen to the concerns of others

_____ 31. The ability to use eye-hand coordination and to work with instrumentation and equipment of various shapes and sizes

True/False

Indicate whether the sentence or statement is true (T) or false (F).

_____ 32. The circulator is considered a sterile team member.

_____ 33. The scrub organizes surgical drapes, instruments, and equipment on the back table.

_____ 34. The scrub may assist in opening a room before performing a surgical scrub.

_____ 35. The surgeon may delegate to the surgical technologist the task of injecting local anesthetics.

_____ 36. The circulator is responsible for documentation of the surgical procedure.

Case Study

Read the following case study and answer the questions based on your knowledge of surgical technology education and certification requirements.

Anne is a 35-year-old female working as a nursing assistant. She is interested in a career change. After considering several allied health careers, Anne became interested in surgical technology. A friend recommended that she visit the Association of Surgical Technologists website to gain further information about the profession. Upon exploring the website, Anne noticed a variety of program options. She learned that it was important to become certified after graduation, and that in order to be eligible to sit for the LCC-ST national certification exam, she would have to attend an accredited program in surgical technology. Anne has applied to a local career college, and if accepted into its surgical technology program, she will graduate with an associate's degree.

1. What is the Association of Surgical Technologists?

_____

_____

2. What are two of Anne's options when choosing a program for her education?

_____

_____

3. Why is becoming certified upon graduation important to surgical technologists?

_____

_____

_____

4. What is the importance of Anne graduating from an accredited program?

_____

_____

_____

5. When Anne graduates and becomes certified, she would be encouraged to maintain continuing education credits. Why is it important for a CST to maintain her or his continuing education credits?

_____

_____

_____

Internet Exercises

1. Enter the key words "Surgical Technology" on a search engine. How many matching websites appeared? What are the top three matching sites?

_____

_____

_____

_____

2. Log onto the ARC-ST website, www.arcst.org, and review the requirements for program accreditation. Then answer the following questions:

    A. How many accredited programs are there in the United States? _____

    B. How many accredited programs are there within your state? _____

    C. How many accredited programs are there within your local area (50-mile radius)? _____

Chapter 2
The Patient

Key Terms

Write the definition for each term.

1. Critical thinking: _____

   _____

2. Direct care: _____

   _____

3. Indirect care: _____

   _____

4. Maslow's hierarchy of needs: _____

   _____

5. Patient-centered care: _____

   _____

6. Therapeutic communication: _____

   _____

Short Answers

7. Explain how the surgical technologist can participate in patient-centered care.

   _____

   _____

   _____

   _____

8. Identify three examples of how a surgical technologist renders direct care to a patient.

   A. _____

   B. _____

   C. _____

9. List three departments or specific personnel involved in indirect care to a patient, and identify a specific task that each may perform.

   A. _____

   _____

   B. _____

   _____

   C. _____

   _____

10. Identify three physiological needs based on Maslow's hierarchy of needs.

   A. _____

   B. _____

   C. _____

11. Which two nutrients are particularly high in demand for the rebuilding of tissues?

   A. _____

   B. _____

Matching

Match each term with the correct definition.

A. food and water

B. esteem need

C. job security

D. paraphrasing

E. direct care

_____ 12. A person's safety needs would include this

_____ 13. "It sounds like you are saying that you are nervous" is an example of this

_____ 14. Applying a dressing to the incision after the case is an example of this

_____ 15. Basic physiological needs are these

_____ 16. Seeking recognition for a job well done is a type of this

True/False

Indicate whether the sentence or statement is true (T) or false (F).

_____ 17. Patient-centered care means that the patient must always be surrounded by nurses, doctors, and other health-care workers.

_____ 18. Therapeutic communication is tailored to each patient.

_____ 19. Toddlers and preschoolers suffer anxiety and fear when separated from their primary caregiver(s).

_____ 20. The patient's spiritual needs are not very important.

_____ 21. Therapeutic communication may be judgmental and condescending to the patient, since the health-care worker knows more than the patient.

Case Studies

Read the following case studies and answer the questions based on your knowledge of surgical technology.

Case 1: You are a patient in Hospital X (use your present age and health status) and have undergone a below-knee amputation of your right leg due to gangrene. Based on Maslow's hierarchy of needs, answer the following questions:

1. Rank the physiological needs that you believe will now be the most difficult to meet first, second, third, and fourth, and explain why.
    Needs include food, water, air, and shelter.

   A. (most difficult) _____

   B. _____

   C. _____

   D. (least difficult) _____

   _____

   _____

   _____

2. Explain how your health-care providers and family can assist you in meeting the need you identified as being the most difficult to meet.

Case 2: Your patient scheduled for surgery in your operating room does not speak English and understands few English words. Describe some therapeutic communication techniques that you could employ to convey caring, support, and empathy to this patient.

Internet Exercise

Log onto www.childhooddevelopmentinfo.com/development/devsequence.shtml. Choose a childhood stage of development, and discuss what to expect of the child you have chosen and how you can effectively communicate with her or him as your surgical patient.

Chapter 3
Law and Ethics

Key Terms

Write the definition for each term.

1. Ethical dilemma: _____

   _____

2. Ethics: _____

   _____

3. Informed consent form: _____

   _____

4. Laws: _____

   _____

5. Liable: _____

   _____

6. Malpractice: _____

   _____

7. Negligence: _____

   _____

8. Sentinel event: _____

   _____

Short Answers

9. Morals may be described as what?

_____

_____

10. Ethics is described as what?

_____

_____

11. Laws are described as what?

_____

_____

12. In the United States, four sources of law regulate society. Identify the four, and briefly describe each.

_____

_____

_____

_____

13. The surgical technologist works under the direct supervision of whom?

_____

_____

14. Under the U.S. Constitution, each state has the power to regulate businesses and professions, including the practice of medicine and professional nursing. The laws differ from state to state and require a person to obtain a license to practice medicine or nursing. What are these laws called?

_____

_____

_____

_____

15. Accredited hospitals and other health-care facilities are required to orient and make available to employees printed documents that detail the policies and procedures required for that facility. Each new employee must become familiar with and understand the procedures that dictate her or his job performance and responsibilities. Why is this important?

_____

_____

_____

_____

16. Name and describe two manuals that are important in the operating room.

_____

_____

17. Define the doctrine of *respondeat superior* liability.

_____

_____

18. A tort is a civil wrong—an act committed against a person or a person's property. Whereas a criminal act can result in a fine or an imprisonment, a civil wrong can result in a lawsuit in which money is rewarded to the injured party. There are two types of torts. Name and briefly describe each.

_____

_____

_____

19. Negligence is considered an unintentional tort; there are many situations in the surgical setting in which negligence on the surgical technologist's part can injure patients and/or coworkers. These injuries can result in lawsuits against STs as well as their employers. List two ways in which STs can avoid these situations.

_____

_____

_____

20. There is no excuse for mistaken identity or for an operation on the wrong side or site or on the wrong patient. How may these mistakes be prevented?

_____

_____

21. The surgical technologist's responsibility in handling specimens requires careful attention. If the specimen is removed to confirm or rule out malignancy, loss or lack of proper labeling can have what consequences?

_____

_____

_____

22. The surgical technologist is not licensed to administer drugs. However, he or she does accept drugs from the circulator. Briefly explain the surgical technologist's responsibility before and during passing these drugs to the surgeon.

_____

_____

23. The Health Insurance and Accountability Act of 1996 (HIPAA) was created by the U.S. Department of Human Services to do what?

_____

_____

24. A patient's operative consent form is a legal document that describes the risks, possible complications, benefits, and nature of a medical procedure, including surgery. The patient has been brought to the operating room, and as the anesthesia provider is speaking to the patient, he or she realizes that the patient does not understand the procedure for which he or she is scheduled. What should be done?

_____

_____

_____

25. Describe an incident report.

_____

_____

26. What is the difference between an advance directive and a living will?

_____

_____

27. Professional organizations, such as the Association of Surgical Technologists, have created codes of ethics that reflect the expectations of professional surgical technologists, as they make decisions involving ethical issues. By acting in accordance with these ethics, STs demonstrate what?

_____

_____

_____

Matching

Match each term with the correct definition.

A. abandonment

B. complaint

C. deposition

D. damages

E. malpractice

F. liable

G. perjury

H. libel

I. sentinel event

J. summons

_____ 28. Testimony of a witness, under oath, and transcribed by a court reporter during the pretrial phase of a civil lawsuit

_____ 29. A court-issued document that is received by a person being sued, notifying the person that he or she is a defendant in the lawsuit

_____ 30. The legal document that begins a civil lawsuit and designates who is suing and why

_____ 31. Negligence committed by a professional. May also be committed when a person deliberately acts outside of her or his scope of practice or while impaired

_____ 32. An unexpected event that occurs; causing death, serious psychological injury, or risk thereof, including any process variation for which a recurrence would carry a significant chance of a serious, adverse outcome

_____ 33. The failure to stay with a patient who is under one's care

_____ 34. Legally responsible and accountable

_____ 35. Money awarded in a civil lawsuit to compensate the injured party

_____ 36. Crime of intentionally lying or falsifying information given during a court testimony after being sworn to tell the truth

_____ 37. Defamation in writing

True/False

Indicate whether the sentence or statement is true (T) or false (F).

_____ 38. To understand the law and how it applies to health care, one must have a basic knowledge of how laws are created and how laws differ from ethics.

_____ 39. A surgical technologist is not directly responsible for his or her actions and cannot be held liable for any acts of negligence, since he or she is a nonlicensed employee.

_____ 40. The hospital manual or orientation manual describes general administrative and logistical issues of the facility. It includes an organizational chart that clarifies the chain of command and information on other topics such as rules pertaining to employee identification privileges and salary procedures.

_____ 41. There are many situations in the surgical setting in which negligence can injure patients or coworkers. Lying about or covering up a surgical count that is not correct at the end of a procedure is not considered a situation that may cause harm to a patient or coworker.

_____ 42. The patient can be seriously and permanently injured because of improper positioning; only those trained and competent to position the patient should perform this task.

Case Studies

Read the following case studies and answer the questions based on your knowledge of law and ethics in the surgical technology field.

Case 1: James is a relatively new surgical technologist. Since passing the national certification exam, he has been working in a large trauma center. He enjoys the fast-paced environment that this type of facility offers. Recently he was the surgical technologist in a trauma case that most of the team members felt was futile. James has been asked to participate in an organ procurement case involving the trauma patient. He is surprised to find out that some of the other team members do not feel that they should be performing some of the procedures that they do.

1. Do you believe that health-care professionals are required to do everything possible to save and/or prolong a patient's life?

_____

_____

2. Describe or define your idea of futile.

_____

_____

3. What do you consider more important, quality or quantity of life? Describe each.

_____

_____

_____

4. Do you believe the patient has the "right to die?" Briefly explain your answer.

_____

_____

_____

5. As a surgical technologist, does James have the right to refuse to participate in certain cases that violate his ethical, moral, or religious values? What was his obligation to the facility regarding this issue when he was hired?

_____

_____

_____

Case 2: Susanne has graduated from an accredited surgical technology program and has passed the national certification exam. She has accepted a job in a local hospital operating room. She has been given her room assignment and introduced to her preceptor, Joanne. While walking to their room, Joanne stops and begins to talk to a group of employees about a patient's medical history, one she had the day before. As they continue on to their room, the preceptor says to Susanne, "Don't tell anyone, but I think Donna is under the influence of drugs or alcohol." Susanne and Joanne are setting up for the case as the anesthesia care provider comes into the room. Joanne makes a lewd comment to him that obviously causes him embarrassment, and this behavior continues throughout the case.

1. What title has Susanne earned by passing the national certification exam?

   _____

2. Did Susanne's preceptor have the right to discuss her patient's medical history with coworkers? Why?

   _____

   _____

   _____

3. What is Joanne's legal and ethical responsibility concerning Donna?

   _____

   _____

   _____

4. By making lewd comments that were embarrassing to the anesthesia care provider and continuing this behavior throughout the case, Joanne is guilty of what? Why is this type of behavior illegal and unethical?

   _____

   _____

   _____

5. Can Susanne refuse to work with Joanne?

   _____

Internet Exercise

Go to the Association for Surgical Technologists (www.ast.org) website and look up the standards of practice listed under education and standards. After reading through the standards of practice, write a short paragraph describing the competencies of the certified surgical technologist at different levels.

   _____

   _____

   _____

   _____

Chapter 4
Hospital Administration and Organization

Key Terms

Write the definition for each term.

1. Accreditation: _____

_____

_____

2. Chain of command: _____

_____

_____

3. JCAHO: _____

_____

_____

4. Mission statement: _____

_____

_____

_____

5. Nonprofit hospital: _____

_____

_____

6. Organizational chart: _____

_____

_____

19

7. OSHA: _____

_____

_____

8. Proprietary hospital: _____

_____

_____

9. Risk management: _____

_____

_____

10. Satellite facilities: _____

_____

Short Answers

11. List three facilities in which surgery can be performed, and give a brief description of the type of procedure that may be performed in each setting.

_____

_____

_____

12. As a surgical technologist working in an operating room, you will work closely with other departments in the hospital. List three ancillary departments that you may work with, and briefly describe how they are associated with the operating room.

_____

_____

_____

13. Surgical technologists function as part of a team. Each team member has his or her own job description. To find a copy of your job description, where would you look?

_____

_____

_____

14. Who or what is the JCAHO?

_____

_____

_____

15. Hospital management and operational staff are usually organized into three separate bodies. Name the three bodies, and describe the responsibilities of each.

_____

_____

_____

16. What does OSHA stand for?

_____

_____

_____

17. Hospitals and health-care facilities have mission statements. What is a mission statement, and what is its purpose?

_____

_____

_____

18. The surgeon requests that the specimen he has removed be sent for a frozen-section analysis. What department will receive the specimen? What steps will be taken to provide the surgeon with an immediate tissue evaluation?

_____

_____

_____

19. The medical records department is responsible for receiving, maintaining, and transferring all patient records. Because patient records are considered legal documents, strict protocols exist regarding when signatures are required, who may make entries, what must be included, and where the patient's documents should be stored. What type of information may be found in the chart?

_____

_____

_____

20. The operative report is filled out by the circulating nurse and signed by members of the operating team. This report becomes the permanent legal record of safety measures taken, the care plan, and any incidents that occurred during surgery. What type of information may be contained in this report?

_____

_____

_____

Matching

Match each term with the correct definition.

A. nonprofit hospital

B. chain of command

C. anesthesiologist

D. risk management

E. certified surgical technologist-certified first assistant (CST/CFA)

_____ 21. Responsible for the meticulous assessment, monitoring, and adjustment of the patient's physiologic status during surgery

_____ 22. Directly assists the surgeon with the operation and is specially trained to handle tissue, to provide exposure using instruments and sutures, and to provide hemostasis

_____ 23. Owned by a private group of individuals, usually a corporation. Any financial gains accrued are reinvested in the facility for improvements and maintenance

_____ 24. A hierarchy of personnel positions that establishes both vertical and horizontal relationships between positions

_____ 25. The process of tracking, evaluating, and studying accidents and incidents to protect patients and employees

True/False

Indicate whether the sentence or statement is true (T) or false (F).

_____ 26. Hospitals are classified by their method of financing, their size, and the populations they serve.

_____ 27. Patience, respect, and professionalism build good interdepartmental relationships and help prevent increased stress and interdepartmental conflict.

_____ 28. Because the operating room and the sterile processing department are separated, one is not dependent upon the other. Communication between these two departments is not important.

_____ 29. Nuclear medicine procedures provide information about the structure and function of all organs in the body.

_____ 30. Blood products may be transfused only after two licensed personnel verify the temperature of the products.

Case Studies

Read the following case studies and answer the questions based on your knowledge of hospital administration and organization in the surgical technology field.

Case 1: Irene is an 87-year-old female patient residing at a local nursing home. She is admitted to the hospital with a fractured hip. Irene has been scheduled for a total hip replacement. This surgical procedure will require the services of several departments in the hospital.

1. As you are setting up for this case, you notice that you are missing several instruments. What department will you call to get the needed instruments?

    _____

    _____

2. Who is responsible for transporting Irene to the operating room? What should be done with her chart?

    _____

    _____

3. Irene is brought into the operating room and the circulator notices that the surgeon is not in the room. How may the circulator contact the surgeon?

    _____

    _____

4. During the surgical procedure the anesthesia provider notices that his or her anesthesia machine is not working properly. What department will be notified to come into the operating room to provide maintenance for this complex piece of equipment?

    _____

    _____

5. Irene will require more than 25 days to recover from her surgery. Which type of facility will she spend this time in?

    _____

    _____

Case 2: Walter has just graduated from a surgical technology program. He has an interview for a surgical technologist position at a newly opened ambulatory surgical center near his home. Before going on his interview, Walter did some research on the facility's status regarding accreditation, and he familiarized himself with its mission statement.

1. What is an ambulatory surgical center?

_____

_____

2. Walter learned that the facility is JCAHO accredited. How will the facility benefit from being accredited?

_____

_____

3. Why would Walter want to know what the facility's mission statement contained?

_____

_____

4. If Walter is hired, what will he gain from reading the facility's policies?

_____

_____

5. After working as a certified surgical technologist (CST), Walter would like to continue his education and become a certified surgical technologist-certified first assistant (CST-CFA). How may he do this?

_____

_____

Internet Exercise

Using the Internet as a tool, research a member of the operating room personnel and write a brief report on his or her education and training requirements.

_____

_____

_____

_____

_____

_____

_____

_____

_____

_____

_____

_____

_____

_____

_____

_____

_____

_____

_____

_____

_____

Chapter 5
Operating Room Environment

Key Terms

Write the definition for each term.

1. Air exchange: _____

_____

_____

2. Case-cart system: _____

_____

_____

3. Central core: _____

_____

_____

4. Contaminated: _____

_____

_____

5. Decontamination area: _____

_____

_____

6. Efficiency: _____

_____

_____

7. High-efficiency particulate air (HEPA) filters: _____

_____

_____

8. Laminar airflow (LAF) system: _____

_____

_____

_____

9. Restricted area: _____

_____

_____

_____

10. Semirestricted area: _____

_____

_____

11. Sterile: _____

_____

_____

12. Traffic flow: _____

_____

_____

13. Transitional area: _____

_____

_____

14. Unrestricted area: _____

_____

Short Answers

15. The operating room design is based on three principles. Name the three principles, and briefly explain each.

_____

_____

_____

_____

16. Many different types of floor plans meet the goals of environmental safety, efficiency, and separation of clean from hazardous or contaminated areas of the department. What is the primary function of the floor plan?

_____

_____

_____

_____

17. Traffic flow is the movement of people and equipment into, out of, and within the operating room. The flow of personnel moves from nonrestricted to restricted areas, as equipment is prepared, transported, and stored; it must follow the same pattern. What is the goal of traffic flow?

_____

_____

_____

_____

18. The locker room is the transitional area for those needing to change into scrub attire. Clean scrub attire must be located in an area protected from contamination by fluids or soil. Explain why head caps should be available in the same area as scrub attire.

_____

_____

_____

_____

19. Semirestricted areas require personnel to don scrub suits and hair caps before entering. Identify two semirestricted areas of the operating room, and briefly describe each.

_____

_____

_____

_____

20. The operating table on which the patient is positioned for surgery is adjustable for height, degree of tilt, orientation in the room, articular breaks, and length. Many accessories are available to meet the needs of different surgical procedures. Identify three operating table accessories, and describe their functions.

_____

_____

_____

_____

21. Many pieces of furniture are standard in surgical suites. They must be made of stainless steel, which is nonporous and easy to decontaminate. Identify and briefly describe the function of three pieces of equipment that you, as a surgical technologist, will use.

_____

_____

_____

_____

22. Airflow from nonrestricted to restricted areas can increase the risk of infection. To decrease this risk, air pressure in the surgical suite is maintained at a level that is 10% higher than the air pressure in adjacent semirestricted areas. Surgical suite doors must remain closed. Why?

_____

_____

_____

_____

23. In the operating room suite, computers are used for patient charting and documentation. Describe another use for computers within the surgical setting.

_____

_____

_____

_____

24. Protection of sensitive information is of the utmost importance in the health-care setting. Safeguards have been put into place to prevent unauthorized access to patient-specific information. Violation of a patient's confidentiality can result in serious sanctions, including termination of employment. What are some security measures that protect the patient's confidentiality?

_____

_____

_____

Matching

Match each term with the correct definition.

A. decontamination area

B. restricted area

C. traffic flow

D. case-cart system

E. efficiency

F. transitional area

G. central core

H. unrestricted area

I. contaminated area

J. semirestricted area

_____ 25. Area where surgical personnel can find scrub attire to change into, where they will prepare to enter the semirestricted or restricted areas

_____ 26. Room or small department where soiled instruments and equipment are cleaned of gross soil and decontaminated

_____ 27. The goal is always to prevent contaminated items from coming into contact with clean and sterile items; the movement of people and equipment into, out of, and within the operating room

_____ 28. The restricted area of the operating room where sterile supplies and flash sterilizers are located

_____ 29. A system of gathering and transporting items needed for surgery

_____ 30. Instruments, supplies, or items that have been exposed to a nonsterile item, particle, or surface through physical or airborne contact

_____ 31. Personnel dressed in street clothes and portable equipment that has not been disinfected are confined to this area

_____ 32. Area where scrub sinks are located, corridors, and equipment and supply rooms

_____ 33. The economic use of time and energy to prevent unnecessary expenditure of work, materials, and time

_____ 34. Area where surgical masks are required

True/False

Indicate whether the sentence or statement is true (T) or false (F).

_____ 35. It is permissible to allow another coworker to use your computer password.

_____ 36. Prep solution should not be stored in a warmer; the heat from the warmer tends to decrease the efficacy of the antibacterial solution.

_____ 37. Temperature control is not an important component of patient care and safety.

_____ 38. Electrical outlets in the operating room must be grounded.

_____ 39. In the event of malfunction or emergency, in-line gas and suction connections may be altered as needed to finish the surgical procedure.

_____ 40. In-line gas is used to provide a power source for drills and other medical devices requiring high-speed operation without the danger of electrical cords on the sterile field.

_____ 41. Suction should not be turned off until the patient leaves the room.

_____ 42. Headlights are worn by many surgeons in case of power failures.

_____ 43. Not all surgery takes place in the operating room. As a surgical technologist, you may be asked to help with a procedure in another department of the facility.

_____ 44. When performing a surgical procedure in another department, the principles of patient care and asepsis do not change, even though the circumstances and location may be different than usual.

Case Studies

Read the following case studies and answer the questions based on your knowledge of the operating room environment in the surgical technology field.

Case 1: This is Eve's big day! She is scrubbing in on her first case as a student. Eve has researched her case and desperately hopes to do everything right.

1. Arriving in street clothes, where will Eve find the proper surgical attire to change into and a place to store her personal belongings?

_____

_____

_____

2. Should Eve store her lunch in her locker? Why?

_____

_____

_____

3. Before Eve can do her surgical scrub, she will need to prepare herself to enter a restricted area. She also will need protective eyewear for the case. What will she need to enter the restricted area? Where will Eve find the items she needs?

_____

_____

_____

4. During the case, Eve has quite a few soiled sponges. Into which piece of equipment should Eve discard the sponges?

_____

_____

_____

5. During the case, Eve notices moisture on the ceiling. What should she do?

_____

_____

_____

Case 2: Rhonda is the circulator in Room 4. The surgeon has just started a hernia repair on the patient, and Rhonda is documenting the operative report on the computer. Sara, another circulator, comes into the room to relieve Rhonda for lunch. As Rhonda starts to log off of the computer, Sara says, "Don't bother with that, I'll just work under your password."

1. Why are computer passwords important?

_____

_____

_____

2. Should Rhonda allow Sara to document under her password? Why?

_____

_____

_____

3. What should Rhonda do before leaving for lunch? Why?

_____

_____

_____

4. Health-care institutions protect patient information by conducting electronic audits. What are electronic audits?

_____

_____

_____

5. If you forget your password, or if your computer access key is lost or stolen, what should you do?

_____

_____

_____

Internet Exercise

Using the Internet as a research tool, research the effects that environmental factors such as temperature, humidity, and air exchange in the OR have on the sterility of instruments and packs.

Chapter 6
Communication and Teamwork

Key Terms

Write the definition for each term.

1. Aggressiveness: _____

_____

_____

2. Assertiveness: _____

_____

_____

3. Consensus: _____

_____

_____

4. Content: _____

_____

_____

5. Feedback: _____

_____

_____

6. Gossip: _____

_____

_____

7. Groupthink: _____

_____

_____

8. Norms: _____

_____

_____

9. Receiver: _____

_____

_____

10. Sender: _____

_____

_____

11. Tone: _____

_____

_____

12. Values: _____

_____

_____

13. Win-Lose: _____

_____

_____

14. Win-Win: _____

_____

_____

Short Answers

15. What is communication?

_____

_____

_____

16. Clear communication clarifies relationships and helps establish professional and social boundaries. It increases teamwork and reinforces team goals. Good communication greatly increases the safety of the environment for the patient. Poor communication will result in what?

_____

_____

_____

17. What are some ways people communicate their needs, ideas, and feelings?

_____

_____

_____

18. The assertive person does not submit to the aggression of others but self-advocates by stating his or her needs clearly, without hesitation or self-effacement. Assertiveness is the ability to do what?

_____

_____

_____

19. People immediately sense when another person respects them. The person's actions and speech clearly show respect. Respect for others communicates recognition of what?

_____

_____

_____

20. Because of the unique environment of the operating room, problem behaviors often lead to open conflict. What are some characteristics of operating room work that contribute to problem behaviors?

_____

_____

_____

21. Verbal abuse has a negative effect on patient care; it causes staff to become tense, upset, and distracted. Verbal abuse affects morale, reduces productivity, and increases errors and staff turnover. Verbal abuse is considered what?

_____

_____

_____

22. These often lead to creative solutions that provide a safer and more efficient operating room, and they are important in creating changed conditions in the workplace. What are they?

_____

23. Gossip is the telling and retelling of events about another's personal life, professional life, or physical condition. A rumor is information, the validity of which is questionable. Both gossip and rumors have damaging effects. An important rule to follow concerning gossip and rumors is what?

_____

_____

_____

24. A team is a group of people coming together to reach common goals. The surgical team includes the surgeon, anesthesia provider, assistants, surgical technologist, and registered nurse/circulator. The qualities of good teamwork are reflected in the team's ability to reach its goals. In providing quality patient care, each member of the surgical team should retain which qualities?

_____

_____

_____

Matching

Match each term with the correct definition.

A. assertiveness

B. win-win

C. norms

D. groupthink

E. win-lose

F. values

G. aggressiveness

H. gossip

I. tone

J. feedback

_____ 25. Reflects the sender's emotions, such as respect for the receiver, opinion about the message, or attitude toward the receiver

_____ 26. The exertion of power over others by intimidation, loudness, or bullying—qualities that ignore others' feelings or take advantage of others' vulnerabilities

_____ 27. The ability to express one's needs and rights while respecting the needs and rights of others

_____ 28. A response to the sender's message

_____ 29. Beliefs, customs, behaviors, and norms that a person defends and upholds

_____ 30. In conflict resolution, a situation in which both parties of conflict gain by the solution

_____ 31. Behaviors that are accepted as part of the environment and culture of a group, usually established by customs and popular acceptance rather than by law

_____ 32. The goal is to shock or evoke intrigue

_____ 33. Collective behavior and thinking

_____ 34. In conflict resolution, one party finds the solution satisfactory, while the other party finds it unsatisfactory

True/False

Indicate whether the sentence or statement is true (T) or false (F).

_____ 35. Participating in the spreading of gossip or rumors in the operating room is an excellent communication skill for the surgical technologist.

_____ 36. Silence and stillness are not considered a method of communication but "dead space" that must be filled with conversation.

_____ 37. People who possess good listening skills are easy to talk to.

_____ 38. Listening does not require participation. Passive listening leads to accurate interpretation and/or the ability to respond to the information.

_____ 39. Conflict in the operating room cannot be managed unless people communicate about their problems.

_____ 40. Setting priorities in the operating room requires the team's consensus, an agreement on what the goals are, and how these goals will be reached.

_____ 41. Sexual harassment is not considered illegal, because the perpetrator usually considers the behavior innocent.

_____ 42. Rude, vulgar, and offensive behavior is not a natural reaction to the stress of the operating room environment. It is a choice made by those who perpetrate it—individuals who use their authority to hurt others.

_____ 43. Because of the intense environment in the operating room, a team member's intensity has no effect on the others.

_____ 44. One of the most important reasons to increase communication skills is to maintain respect, trust, and empathy among coworkers and management.

Case Studies

Read the following case studies and answer the questions based on your knowledge of communication and teamwork in the surgical technology field.

Case 1: It is your first day of orientation at your new job. You have graduated from an accredited surgical technology program with an associate's degree and have successfully passed the certification exam giving you the right to use the title "Certified Surgical Technologist." The OR educator introduces you to several of the employees, including your preceptor. Later at the scrub sink, your preceptor says to you "No one here is going to accept you; we have all been trained on the job and know exactly what is expected of us. Why would you want to waste your time going to school for this type of employment?"

1. How would you handle this situation?

_____

_____

_____

_____

Case 2: The surgical technology students from the local community college would like to nominate Blaine Smith, surgical technologist, from the operating room, for the Communication and Teamwork Award. Blaine has gone above and beyond expectations in teaching students. He makes a special effort to teach students during the operative procedure, as well as to keep his intensity and focus on the patient and procedure. Blaine's personal attention to each student and her or his personality has been very much appreciated. His ability to communicate on a professional basis with both the students and the other surgical team members is remarkable. He has been mentioned a number of times by surgical technology students as the "number-1 preceptor" to work with. His dedication to teaching and his personality have made him the nominee for the Communication and Teamwork Award. Using communication and teamwork skills as a basis, write a short paragraph on the qualities you feel would make a number-1 preceptor.

_____

_____

_____

_____

_____

Internet Exercise

Consider the incidence of wrong-site surgery. The Joint Commission on Accreditation of Healthcare Organizations (JCAHO) recently published a sentinel event alert regarding significant concerns related to wrong-site surgery. This report is a follow-up to an August 1998 alert regarding the same problem. The recent report addresses concerns that, despite national attention and efforts by professional associations and regulatory groups, the incidence of wrong-site surgery remains extremely high. The JCAHO reports that in the majority of cases, communication breaks down between surgical team members, the patient, and his or her family members.

Wrong-site surgery is just one way that poor communication and lack of teamwork affect patient care in the operating room. Using the Internet as a research tool, write a brief paragraph on other ways the patient is affected by the communication and teamwork skills of those employed in the operating room.

_____

_____

_____

_____

_____

_____

_____

_____

_____

Chapter 7
Microbiology and the Process of Infection

Key Terms

Write the definition for each term.

1. Acquired immunity: _____

   _____

   _____

2. Aerosol droplet: _____

   _____

   _____

3. Antibiotic resistant: _____

   _____

   _____

4. Antibodies: _____

   _____

   _____

5. Antigens: _____

   _____

   _____

6. Bacteria (pl); Bacterium (sing): _____

   _____

   _____

7. Colonization: _____

_____

_____

8. Convalescence: _____

_____

_____

9. Cross-contamination: _____

_____

_____

10. Dehiscence: _____

_____

_____

11. Direct transmission: _____

_____

_____

12. Droplet nuclei: _____

_____

_____

13. Endospore (spore): _____

_____

_____

14. Endotoxin: _____

_____

_____

15. Evisceration: _____

_____

_____

16. Exotoxin: _____

_____

_____

17. Fomite: _____

_____

_____

18. Gram stain: _____

_____

_____

19. Host: _____

_____

_____

20. Indirect transmission: _____

_____

_____

21. Infection: _____

_____

_____

22. Inflammation: _____

_____

_____

23. Innate immunity: _____

_____

_____

24. Nonpathogenic: _____

_____

25. Nosocomial infection: _____

_____

_____

26. Obligate aerobe: _____

_____

_____

27. Obligate anaerobe: _____

_____

_____

28. Parasite: _____

_____

_____

29. Pathogens: _____

_____

_____

30. Phagocyte: _____

_____

_____

31. Portal of entry: _____

_____

_____

32. Prion: _____

_____

_____

33. Prodromal: _____

_____

_____

34. Prokaryote: _____

_____

_____

35. Reservoir: _____

_____

_____

36. Resident microorganisms: _____

_____

_____

37. Retrovirus: _____

_____

_____

38. Standard precautions: _____

_____

_____

39. Transient microorganisms: _____

_____

_____

40. Transmission: _____

_____

_____

41. Vector: _____

_____

_____

42. Virulence: _____

_____

_____

43. Virus: _____

_____

_____

Short Answers

44. Disease is a state of altered health. There are many different sources of disease, such as genetic mutation, the environment, and stress. The disease can be localized or systemic. Define localized and systemic.

_____

_____

_____

45. When organisms of two different species live together, it is called _____. If neither organism is harmed, it is referred to as _____; if the association is of benefit to both, it is _____; and if one is harmed and the other benefits, it is _____.

_____

_____

_____

46. The binomial classification system differentiates microorganisms (microscopic entities that reproduce independently of a host) into two groups, prokaryotes and eukaryotes. Define each.

_____

_____

_____

47. The types of microbes that cause most infectious diseases that affect humans are called what?

_____

_____

_____

48. Bacteria are partially identified by their structure. The study of form and structure is referred to as morphology. There are three separate forms or shapes of bacteria. Identify the three shapes of bacteria, and give one example of pathogenic disease caused by each.

_____

_____

_____

49. Important environmental parameters for bacteria reproduction include what?

_____

_____

_____

50. Oxygen requirements for bacteria vary widely. A microorganism that needs oxygen to live and grow is called what? A microorganism that does not require oxygen for reproduction is called what?

_____

_____

_____

51. *Staphylococcus aureus* is the most widespread cause of surgical site infections. It is gram-positive resident bacteria of the skin transmitted to the surgical site wound by direct or indirect contact with a health-care worker, a contaminated object, or another patient. Name two antibiotic-resistant strains of *S. aureus* and the antibiotic to which each is resistant.

_____

_____

_____

52. Blood-borne pathogens are a direct threat to hospitalized patients and all health-care personnel. Because of the high risk of transmission through contact with blood and body fluids, the CDC has developed strict protocols for handling patients, medical waste, body fluids, and soiled equipment. These protocols are called what?

_____

_____

_____

53. The care of individuals stricken with HIV requires our utmost ethical and humanitarian consideration. To give less is to deny our commitment to the suffering of all people, regardless of the nature or cause of that suffering. HIV is transmitted via what?

_____

_____

_____

Matching

Match each term with the correct definition.

A. hepatitis

B. Creutzfeldt-Jakob disease (CJD)

C. fungi

D. protozoal diseases

E. arthropods

F. infectious process

G. vector

H. fomite

I. respiratory transmission

J. innate immunity

_____ 54. Depends on many conditions, including physiologic and immunologic integrity of the host, the dose of invading organisms, and the microorganism's ability to resist or debilitate the body's defenses

_____ 55. Generally associated with public health conditions such as dirty water, improper sanitation, and inattention to food safety

_____ 56. A disease of the liver that is caused by one of three significant viruses

_____ 57. Carry very small bacteria called rickettsias

_____ 58. Present from birth, but can be affected by health status, age, and genetics

_____ 59. An inanimate object that is capable of harboring and transmitting disease

_____ 60. Current infection control standards require the use of disposable instruments or specialized decontamination procedures

_____ 61. Found worldwide on living organic substances, in water, and in soil and classified into two groups, molds and yeasts

_____ 62. A living organism carrying pathogenic microorganisms from one source to another

_____ 63. Occurs by an aerosol droplet when microorganisms are transmitted from the respiratory tract of one person to another after water droplets are forcefully expelled during talking, coughing, or sneezing

True/False

Indicate whether the sentence or statement is true (T) or false (F).

_____ 64. Shortly after birth, an infant's body begins to acquire a wide variety of bacterial colonies that exists in symbiosis with the host within certain tissues of the body. These are called normal or resident flora.

_____ 65. Microorganisms that come into contact with the body and remain are called transient microorganisms.

_____ 66. Intact skin, including the mucous membranes, provides an excellent barrier against the transmission and spread of infection.

_____ 67. Skin appendages such as the eyelashes and nasal and ear hair prevent contamination by dust and droplets.

_____ 68. Primary defenses in the gastrointestinal tract do not include normal bacterial flora.

_____ 69. In phagocytosis, a response of the lymphatic system to inflammation, specialized leukocytes rush to the site of the foreign pathogen, bind to the wall of the microorganism, and then surround and engulf it.

_____ 70. Active immunity occurs when the body receives the specific disease antibodies from an outside source.

_____ 71. There are no strains of pathogens that are resistant to, or partially resistant to, the most powerful antimicrobial agents available.

_____ 72. The general preoperative condition of the patient may directly affect factors influencing the extent and severity of surgical site infections.

_____ 73. A surgical site infection can be fatal.

Case Study

Read the following case study and answer the question based on your knowledge of microbiology and the process of infection in the surgical technology field.

The incidence of nosocomial or hospital-acquired infections is about 5 to 10%. Hospital infection control programs can prevent 33% of nosocomial infections. The mechanism of action of nosocomial infection, as in any other infectious disease, is dependent on host, agent, and environmental factors. Risk factors for the host are age, nutritional status, and coexisting disorders. A nosocomial infection is influenced by the microbe's intrinsic virulence as well as its ability to colonize and survive within institutions. Diagnostic procedures, medical devices, and medical and surgical treatment are risk factors in the hospital environment.

1. As a surgical technologist, it is important for you to know and use standard precautions to protect yourself and the patient. Describe standard precautions.

   _____

   _____

   _____

   _____

Internet Exercise

Using the Internet as a research tool, write a brief paragraph about stress and its relationship to disease.

_____

_____

_____

_____

_____

_____

_____

Chapter 8

Disinfection, Decontamination, and Sterilization Standards and Practices

Key Terms

Write the definition for each term.

1. Antisepsis: _____

_____

_____

2. Bactericidal: _____

_____

_____

3. Bacteriostatic: _____

_____

_____

4. Bioburden: _____

_____

_____

5. Biological indicator: _____

_____

_____

6. Cavitation: _____

_____

_____

7. Chemical indicator: _____

_____

_____

8. Chemical sterilization: _____

_____

_____

9. Cleaning: _____

_____

_____

10. Cobalt 60 radiation: _____

_____

_____

11. Critical items: _____

_____

_____

12. Decontamination: _____

_____

_____

13. Disinfection: _____

_____

_____

14. Ethylene oxide: _____

_____

_____

15. Event-related sterility: _____

_____

_____

16. Fungicidal: _____

_____

_____

17. Germicidal: _____

_____

_____

18. Gravity displacement sterilizer: _____

_____

_____

19. High-level disinfection: _____

_____

_____

20. High-vacuum sterilizer: _____

_____

_____

21. Inanimate: _____

_____

_____

22. Lumen: _____

_____

_____

23. Noncritical items: _____

_____

_____

24. Peracetic acid: _____

_____

_____

25. Plasma sterilization: _____

_____

_____

26. Sanitation: _____

_____

_____

27. Semicritical items: _____

_____

_____

28. Shelf life: _____

_____

_____

29. Sporicidal: _____

_____

_____

30. Sterilization: _____

_____

_____

31. Ultrasonic cleaner: _____

_____

_____

32. Virucidal: _____

_____

_____

33. Washer-sterilizer: _____

_____

_____

Short Answers

34. Identify and briefly describe the three categories of classifying patient-care equipment commonly disinfected or sterilized in the health-care setting.

_____

_____

_____

35. Factors that affect a disinfectant's activity or ability include what?

_____

_____

_____

36. Because of the toxicity of some disinfectants, precautions should always be used when working with these chemicals. List three precautions when working with disinfectants.

_____

_____

_____

37. An important step in the decontamination of the surgical suite is done before the workday begins. Explain what should be done in the surgical suite before the beginning of the workday, and why.

_____

_____

_____

38. The most common method used to decontaminate stainless steel surgical instruments is the washer-sterilizer. The washer-sterilizer not only cleans but also sterilizes the instruments. Explain how the washer-sterilizer operates.

_____

_____

_____

39. Define sterility, and explain the importance of sterility in the operating room.

_____

_____

_____

40. Briefly explain the use of a flash sterilizer in the operating room.

_____

_____

_____

41. Subjecting items to the process of sterilization does not ensure that they are sterile. Objective testing or monitoring is needed to verify both the mechanical process and outcome. Describe one way to verify that the sterilization method has effectively destroyed all microorganisms.

_____

_____

_____

42. After an item is processed and sterilized, consideration must be given to how the item can be kept sterile. Time-related sterility measures, which are based on the period of time since sterilization, are no longer commonly used. Event-related sterility or terminal sterilization is the accepted standard. Explain event-related sterility.

_____

_____

_____

Matching

Match each term with the correct definition.

A. critical items

B. cavitation

C. sporicidal

D. inanimate

E. event-related sterility

F. lumen

G. bioburden

H. decontamination

I. antisepsis

J. sterilization

_____ 43. The debris and microorganisms that contaminate an item

_____ 44. A process in which all types of microorganisms, including spores, are destroyed

_____ 45. Used by the ultrasonic cleaner, a process in which air pockets are imploded, releasing particles of soil and tissue debris from instruments

_____ 46. The inside portion of a hollow tube or instrument

_____ 47. Includes vascular and urinary catheters, implants, surgical instruments, and needles

_____ 48. Highly effective against all types of microbes and said to achieve a high level of disinfection

_____ 49. Nonliving, not alive

_____ 50. To render the operating room environment, which includes all cleanable surfaces as disease-free as possible

_____ 51. A process that destroys most pathogenic organisms on animate surfaces

_____ 52. Sterilized items are assumed sterile between uses, unless the environmental condition or integrity of the package has been compromised

True/False

Indicate whether the sentence or statement is true (T) or false (F).

_____ 53. An instrument that is dropped during a surgical procedure and is needed to complete the procedure may be flash sterilized.

_____ 54. It is safe to consider items sterile by simply placing them into a sterilizer and running it for the required amount of time.

_____ 55. Disinfection is a process by which all pathogenic microorganisms on animate surfaces are destroyed.

_____ 56. Personal protective equipment includes protective eyewear, gloves, mask, and cover gown.

_____ 57. Standard precautions must be carried out to prevent cross-contamination with blood-borne pathogens.

_____ 58. During surgery, it is each team member's responsibility to ensure that the environment of the surgical suite is kept as disease-free as possible.

_____ 59. It is acceptable for the circulator to line up dirty sponges on the floor for counting.

_____ 60. It is not necessary for the surgical technologist to keep instruments flushed and wiped of tissue and blood during the surgical procedure.

_____ 61. Any instrument exposed to the sterile field must go through the terminal processing steps, whether it appears soiled or not.

_____ 62. The case-cart system is used to transport clean items for surgery from the outside department and contaminated items from the surgery back to the appropriate department.

Case Studies

Read the following case studies and answer the questions based on your knowledge of disinfection, decontamination, and sterilization standards and practices in the surgical technology field.

Case 1: Sanitation practices should aim to provide a clean environment for the perioperative patient and be carried out in a manner that poses minimal risk of exposure to infectious waste to the patient as well as to the surgical team. The circulator's task is to keep the OR orderly during surgery, including spot cleaning any contamination of blood or bodily fluids with a hospital-grade germicide, to maintain a sterile field, to keep the floor clean, and to use the proper receptacles for waste. Other sanitation responsibilities in between cases in the OR include ensuring the disposal of sharps in the appropriate containers, removing instruments to appropriate locations on the case cart, suctioning all contaminated fluids into the closed-suction system, removing all drapes and linen used during the procedure, and segregating the materials according to red-bag waste criteria.

1. Describe how the room should be cleaned between each surgical case.

   _____

   _____

   _____

   _____

2. Describe terminal cleaning.

   _____

   _____

   _____

   _____

3. What considerations should be taken in the perimeter area of the operating room?

   _____

   _____

   _____

   _____

Case 2: The Association of Surgical Technologists' description of role definitions and qualifications for the surgical technologist states: "The surgical technologist works under medical supervision to facilitate the safe and effective conduct of invasive surgical procedures. This individual works under the supervision of a surgeon to ensure that the operating room or environment is safe, that equipment functions properly, and that the operative procedure is conducted under conditions that maximize patient safety." A surgical technologist possesses expertise in the theory and application of sterile and aseptic technique and combines the knowledge of human anatomy, surgical procedures, and the implementation of tools and technologies to facilitate a physician's performance of invasive therapeutic and diagnostic procedures.

1. The surgical technologist maintains the neatness of his or her sterile field. When throwing off soiled sponges, where should they be thrown?

2. The circulator is opening a pack of sheets for you, and you notice water spots on the paper. The pack of sheets is contaminated. Explain why the pack is contaminated.

3. During the surgical procedure, it is important to keep instruments wiped of blood and tissue and the lumens of instruments flushed. Why is this important?

4. Can saline be used to clean the instruments? Why?

5. You have dropped an instrument while setting up for a case; you know that the surgeon will want that particular instrument for the case. What will you do?

_____

_____

_____

Internet Exercise

Using the Internet as a research tool, write a brief paragraph explaining the special attention that would be paid to a surgical suite where a patient with tuberculosis will undergo a surgical procedure.

_____

_____

_____

_____

_____

_____

_____

Chapter 9
Aseptic Technique

Key Terms

Write the definition for each term.

1. Airborne contamination: _____

   _____

   _____

2. Antiseptics: _____

   _____

   _____

3. Asepsis: _____

   _____

   _____

4. Aseptic technique: _____

   _____

   _____

5. Chemical barrier: _____

   _____

   _____

6. Closed gloving: _____

   _____

   _____

7. Contamination: _____

_____

_____

8. Hand washing: _____

_____

_____

9. Latex allergy: _____

_____

_____

10. Nonsterile personnel: _____

_____

_____

11. Open gloving: _____

_____

_____

12. Pathogenic: _____

_____

_____

13. Physical barrier: _____

_____

_____

14. Resident flora: _____

_____

_____

15. Scrub: _____

_____

_____

16. Scrubbed personnel: _____

_____

_____

17. Sharps: _____

_____

_____

18. Spatial relations: _____

_____

_____

19. Sterile field: _____

_____

_____

20. Sterile item: _____

_____

_____

21. Sterility: _____

_____

_____

22. Strike-through contamination: _____

_____

_____

23. Surgical conscience: _____

_____

_____

24. Surgical hand scrub: _____

_____

_____

25. Surgical-site infection (SSI): _____

_____

_____

26. Surgically clean: _____

_____

_____

27. Topical antiseptics (antimicrobials): _____

_____

_____

28. Transient flora: _____

_____

_____

Short Answers

29. Give two examples of the application of aseptic technique.

_____

_____

_____

_____

30. Give three examples of important activities and environmental controls that promote and maintain asepsis.

_____

_____

_____

_____

31. An item is sterile or not sterile—the term *sterile* is absolute. Once an item is sterilized, how is its sterility maintained?

_____

_____

_____

_____

32. Why is aseptic technique maintained in cases of gross contamination?

_____

_____

_____

_____

33. Aseptic technique is based on surgical conscience. Explain surgical conscience.

_____

_____

_____

_____

34. Back table covers, Mayo stand covers, and surgical drapes all separate what?

_____

_____

_____

_____

35. Surgical personnel should maintain good personal hygiene habits. List three habits that are important in the surgical setting.

_____

_____

_____

_____

36. Jewelry of any kind is a potential source of pathogens. Surgical personnel must remove all rings, bracelets, and wristwatches. Why is removing all jewelry the recommended standard?

_____

_____

_____

_____

37. Describe how scrub attire should be worn.

_____

_____

_____

_____

38. Before the wrapper of any sterile item is opened, it should be inspected for contamination. Tears, holes, wear marks, or water spots are signs of questionable sterility. What should be done if package sterility is questionable?

_____

_____

_____

_____

Matching

Match each term with the correct definition.

A. latex allergy

B. closed gloving

C. sterile field

D. surgically clean

E. transient flora

F. spatial relations

G. contamination

H. chemical barrier

I. open gloving

J. sharps

_____ 39. A term referring to an awareness of sterile and nonsterile areas or surfaces and one's physical relation to the area or surface

_____ 40. The draped patient is the center; sterile personnel and draped equipment are arranged near the draped patient. Defined by the area or space between sterile personnel and equipment

_____ 41. The sterile glove is protected from the nonsterile hand by the cuff of a surgical gown

_____ 42. Can cause itching, rhinitis, conjunctivitis, and anaphylactic shock, leading to death

_____ 43. Result of physical contact between a sterile surface and a nonsterile surface in surgery

_____ 44. Microorganisms that do not normally reside on the tissue of an individual

_____ 45. The hands and forearms of the person after performance of a surgical scrub

_____ 46. Formed by the action of an antiseptic that not only reduces the number of microorganisms on a surface but also prevents recolonization

_____ 47. Drill bits, trocars, and any item that can easily cause injury

_____ 48. A method generally used when a health-care worker does not wear a sterile gown

True/False

Indicate whether the sentence or statement is true (T) or false (F).

_____ 49. When removing sterile attire contaminated with patient fluids, the gown is removed first.

_____ 50. Unless the surgical technologist is double gloved, he or she must be gloved by another team member, should he or she need to be regloved during a surgical procedure.

_____ 51. When gloving another team member, the glove is oriented so that the palm faces you. Offer the left glove first, and then the right.

_____ 52. Interaction among surgical team members during the process of gowning and gloving often sets the tone for the entire surgical procedure.

_____ 53. As the surgical technologist, you will gown and glove other team members. The preferred order in which to gown and glove team members is to make sure that the CST-CFA has his or her towel, gown, and gloves first, then the surgeon.

_____ 54. The open-gloving technique is used during sterile procedures that do not require donning a sterile gown.

_____ 55. Double gloving is important in reducing the risk of glove failure. To reduce constriction when double gloving, the first or innermost pair of gloves should usually be one size larger than what is normally worn.

_____ 56. When performing your surgical scrub, you must start at the elbows and work toward the fingertips.

_____ 57. The surgical technologist must gown and glove herself or himself from the back table.

_____ 58. Concerning the sterility of an item, when in doubt, throw it out.

Case Studies

Read the following case studies and answer the questions based on your knowledge of aseptic technique in the surgical technology field.

Case 1: Alex is the surgical technologist who is setting up the room for an emergency appendectomy. He is rushing, because he knows the patient will be brought to the room soon. As he takes instruments from a container on his back table to place on his Mayo stand, Alex notices that there is no sterile indicator in the instrument container.

1. Which ethical motivation will Alex use to determine his course of action?

_____

_____

_____

2. What possible risk is Alex posing to the patient if he makes the wrong decision?

_____

_____

_____

3. Alex knows that it will take a few extra minutes to gather the needed supplies to replace his contaminated setup. He is sure that the rest of the team will not be happy about this delay. Why should the rest of the team's happiness not be a concern to Alex right now?

_____

_____

_____

_____

Case 2: According to a clinical report, *Infection Control Today (ICT)* claims that malpractice lawsuits stemming from infection control issues are rare, however, they do occur. Although some patient infections may result despite strict conformity to aseptic technique, only proof of deviation from those standards will support claims of malpractice. The majority of infection-control types of cases are tort (negligence), relying on the showing of negligence (breach of duty) or on *res ipsa loquitur* ("the thing speaks for itself"), a doctrine designed to substitute for the showing of actual negligence.

1. Do you feel that by not following the rules of asepsis, a surgical technologist is guilty of negligence?

_____

_____

_____

2. What are some ways that you personally would be responsible for not promoting and maintaining asepsis?

_____

_____

_____

3. Of all the responsibilities that a surgical technologist may have during his or her career, the most important will always be the guarantor of sterile technique in the operating room. It is your first day at your new job. As the day goes on, you notice that your preceptor's sterile technique is poor; you have seen the preceptor contaminate many things. What will you do?

_____

_____

_____

4. In a lawsuit, is the surgical technologist responsible for his or her own actions? Explain your answer.

_____

_____

_____

Internet Exercise

Cloth hats are a popular alternative to the disposable OR hats offered by health-care facilities for employees. Using the Internet as a research tool, write a brief paragraph on why wearing cloth hats is not always the best choice for OR employees.

_____

_____

_____

_____

_____

_____

Chapter 10
Transporting, Transferring, and Positioning

Key Terms

Write the definition for each term.

1. Abduction: _____

_____

_____

2. Embolism: _____

_____

_____

3. Fowler position: _____

_____

_____

4. Hyperextension: _____

_____

_____

5. Hyperflexion: _____

_____

_____

6. Ischemia: _____

_____

_____

73

7. Jackknife or Kraske position: _____

_____

_____

8. Lateral position: _____

_____

_____

9. Lithotomy position: _____

_____

_____

10. Log roll: _____

_____

_____

11. Necrosis: _____

_____

_____

12. Neuropathy: _____

_____

_____

13. Prone position: _____

_____

_____

14. Reverse Trendelenburg position: _____

_____

_____

15. Semi-Fowler position: _____

_____

_____

16. Shear injury: _____

_____

_____

17. Supine position: _____

_____

_____

18. Table break: _____

_____

_____

19. Thoracic outlet syndrome: _____

_____

_____

20. Thromboembolus: _____

_____

_____

21. Traction injury: _____

_____

_____

22. Transfer board: _____

_____

_____

23. Trendelenburg position: _____

_____

_____

Short Answers

24. Health-care workers are at high risk for back and other types of musculoskeletal injuries while caring for, moving, and transferring patients. How can injuries be reduced?

_____

_____

_____

_____

25. Patient identity is a critical issue in patient care. It is the responsibility of the health-care worker to identify the patient using a standard policy. No patient should be transported until the protocol for proper identification has been completed. What are some appropriate ways to verify patient identification?

_____

_____

_____

_____

26. In the ambulatory care setting, patients walk or are transported by wheelchair to the surgical area. What are three things that can be done to assist a falling patient?

_____

_____

_____

_____

27. When moving a patient to the OR bed from a stretcher, it is important to do what with the stretcher before transferring the patient?

_____

_____

_____

_____

28. Identify three concepts that influence the choice of a surgical position for any given procedure.

_____

_____

_____

_____

29. Identify three correct techniques to follow when positioning the patient.

_____

_____

_____

_____

30. The operating table is used for most operative procedures. It can be configured into many positions and accommodates accessories to aid in maintaining those positions. The perineal cutout allows unrestricted access to what area when the patient is in which position?

_____

_____

_____

_____

31. The supine position, or dorsal recumbent position, is used for procedures of the abdomen, thorax, and face and in orthopedic and vascular surgery. Briefly describe how the patient will be positioned and the positioning aids used to maintain the patient in this position.

_____

_____

_____

_____

32. What are some safety precautions to take when positioning a patient?

_____

_____

_____

_____

33. Shearing causes blood clots and tissue death. Tissue damage that begins as a shearing injury can easily progress to a pressure ulcer. Describe what can happen as pressure on the ulcer causes continued breakdown until the bone is exposed.

_____

_____

_____

_____

Matching

Match each term with the correct definition.

A. abduction

B. hyperextension

C. necrosis

D. thromboembolus

E. log roll

F. thoracic outlet syndrome

G. ischemia

H. hyperflexion

I. neuropathy

J. embolism

_____ 34. Loss of blood supply to a body part, either by compression or blockage within the blood vessels

_____ 35. Obstruction or occlusion of a blood vessel by a blood clot, or trapped air that migrates through the systemic circulation

_____ 36. A technique of moving the patient in which the patient is rolled onto his or her side using a bedsheet or draw sheet

_____ 37. Tissue death

_____ 38. A blood clot that breaks loose and enters the systemic circulation, causing obstruction or occlusion of a blood vessel

_____ 39. Movement of a joint or body part away from the body

_____ 40. Flexion of a joint beyond its normal anatomical range

_____ 41. Permanent or temporary nerve injury that results in numbness or loss of the function of a body part

_____ 42. Extension of a joint beyond its normal anatomical range

_____ 43. A group of disorders attributed to compression of the subclavian vessels and nerves

True/False

Indicate whether the sentence or statement is true (T) or false (F).

_____ 44. Leaving the patient unattended on a stretcher, in a wheelchair, or on an OR bed is abandonment.

_____ 45. It is the responsibility of the health-care employee to verify the patient's identity before transporting him or her.

_____ 46. If the patient has no identification band, it is okay to transport her or him to the OR and provide her or him with an identification band there.

_____ 47. When you are moving a patient it is not necessary to maintain the patient's dignity by keeping him or her covered.

_____ 48. Using a transfer board can help prevent shear injury.

_____ 49. When moving a patient from the OR table to her or his stretcher, the surgeon is at the head of the bed protecting the airway.

_____ 50. Whether the patient is conscious or unconscious, the same precautions are used when moving her or him from the OR table to the stretcher after surgery.

_____ 51. A small child is treated no differently than an adult in the operating room.

_____ 52. Knowledge of anatomy, physiology, and an individual's specific medical condition is not important for patient safety during positioning.

_____ 53. Toboggans, shoulder braces, and stirrups are all accessories used in positioning the patient for surgery.

Case Study

Read the following case study and answer the questions based on your knowledge of transporting, transferring, and positioning in the surgical technology field.

Lewis underwent abdominal surgery to repair a hiatal hernia. He was positioned on the operating table with both of his arms extending outward from each side of the operating table on armboards. The surgeon stood at his right side throughout the procedure, which lasted 1 hour and 20 minutes. When Lewis got to his room afterward, he reported numbness and tingling in his right hand. This persisted well past his discharge from the hospital. Lewis later underwent outpatient nerve conduction studies, which revealed an ulnar nerve injury that did not respond to physical therapy. Tests ruled out other causes for the condition besides injury in the operating room. A procedure was done to reposition the ulnar nerve, which was only partially successful in relieving the numbness and tingling and in restoring function to the injured arm.

1. What would have been the proper positioning for Lewis's arms?

_____

2. What most likely was the cause of Lewis's injury?

_____

3. If you were the surgical technologist for this case and you noticed that the patient's arms were not positioned properly, what would have been your responsibility?

_____

_____

Internet Exercise

Pediatric patients are not "little adults." They require special care in the surgical setting. Using the Internet as a research tool, write a brief paragraph on how the pediatric patient is taken care of in the operating room.

_____

_____

_____

_____

_____

Chapter 11
Surgical Preparation and Draping

Key Terms

Write the definition for each term.

1. Antiseptics: _____

   _____

   _____

2. Barrier drape: _____

   _____

   _____

3. Debridement: _____

   _____

   _____

4. Desiccation: _____

   _____

   _____

5. Drape: _____

   _____

   _____

6. Fenestrated drapes: _____

   _____

   _____

7. Head drape: _____

_____

_____

8. Impervious: _____

_____

_____

9. Incise drapes: _____

_____

_____

10. Prep: _____

_____

_____

11. Residual activity: _____

_____

_____

12. Retention catheter: _____

_____

_____

13. Skin preparation sponge: _____

_____

_____

14. Sterile field: _____

_____

_____

15. Straight catheter: _____

_____

_____

16. Surgical site infection (SSI): _____

_____

_____

Short Answers

17. What is the body's primary defense against infection?

_____

_____

_____

_____

18. What is the most common cause of surgical site infection?

_____

_____

_____

_____

19. Identify and briefly describe three things that may be a part of the patient's preoperative preparation.

_____

_____

_____

_____

20. List one risk to the patient, addressing each part of the preoperative preparation procedure, if the procedure is not performed correctly.

_____

_____

_____

_____

21. Describe surgical skin prep and when it is performed.

_____

_____

_____

_____

22. Most surgical preparation agents are not safe for ophthalmic surgery. List one that can be used for ophthalmic procedures and describe.

_____

_____

_____

_____

23. Identify and describe one patient risk related to surgical prepping.

_____

_____

_____

_____

24. A trauma patient undergoing multiple procedures during one surgery will need what kind of skin preparation?

_____

_____

_____

_____

25. When prepping tissue that is suspected to be cancerous, why is the area prepped differently?

_____

_____

_____

_____

26. Explain the use of towels in the draping procedure.

_____

_____

_____

_____

Matching

Match each term with the correct definition.

A. barrier drapes

B. preparation sponge

C. desiccation

D. impervious

E. prep

F. residual activity

G. incise drapes

H. fenestrated drapes

I. retention catheter

J. straight catheter

_____ 27. Placed in the patient prior to surgical preparation to continuously drain the bladder during surgery

_____ 28. Intended to separate a contaminated area from the incision site

_____ 29. The microbial activity that remains after an antiseptic or a disinfectant has dried

_____ 30. Plastic self-adhesive drape that is placed over the incision site following the surgical prep

_____ 31. A nonradiological detectable sponge

_____ 32. The drying of tissue

_____ 33. Sterile body sheets with a hole or window that exposes the surgical incision site

_____ 34. The use of antiseptic solutions for cleaning the surgical site or a sterile noninvasive procedure such as urinary catheterization

_____ 35. A nonretention catheter used to drain the bladder just before surgery

_____ 36. Not able to be penetrated

True/False

Indicate whether the sentence or statement is true (T) or false (F).

_____ 37. When removing drapes, pull them slowly from the patient, starting at the patient's head and proceeding downward.

_____ 38. The head drape is used for procedures of the nose and throat. It protects the eyes during surgery and provides a sterile barrier over the head.

_____ 39. A patient in the lithotomy position is often awake during the surgical procedure. Always respect the patient's modesty. Do not expose the patient unnecessarily.

_____ 40. Prep and draping of an extremity can safely be done by one person.

_____ 41. When securing towels while draping the patient, always use penetrating towel clips.

_____ 42. Once a sterile drape has been placed, it should not be moved.

_____ 43. A sterile drape that has been placed on the patient is considered completely sterile except for 6 inches up from the floor.

_____ 44. The specific drapes used and the order in which they are applied vary according to the procedure involved, the rules of asepsis, and the surgeon's preference.

_____ 45. An eye drape would not be considered a fenestrated drape.

_____ 46. It is acceptable to use "disposable gloves" and ray-tec sponges for the surgical prep.

Case Studies

Read the following case studies and answer the questions based on your knowledge of surgical preparation and draping in the surgical technology field.

Case 1: Advances in the materials used for disposable and reusable drapes eliminate the need for multiple layers. It is now possible to square off and then use one key drape and/or universal drape of the appropriate reinforcement.

1. What is meant by "squaring off"?

   _____

   _____

   _____

   _____

2. List and briefly describe several ways in which surgical site infections can be avoided in the operating room.

   _____

   _____

   _____

   _____

3. When draping a patient for a surgical procedure, it is important that the drape provide a moisture barrier between the patient and the sterile field. Explain why this is important.

   _____

   _____

   _____

   _____

4. Describe an incise drape and its use.

_____

_____

_____

_____

5. List the different types of procedure drapes and their uses.

_____

_____

_____

_____

Case 2: Despite a great deal of care and concern by medical, nursing, surgical, and engineering personnel, patients continue to suffer inadvertent skin injury in the operating room. Such injuries can prolong morbidity and extend hospitalization, increasing medical costs to the patient and the hospital. The hospital and surgical team also may face liability costs if the injured patient or family sues.

1. Name one prep solution, and describe the type of skin injury that it can cause the surgical patient.

_____

_____

_____

_____

2. How can chemical burns from surgical prep agents be avoided?

_____

_____

_____

_____

3. A patient also can be burned by fire during a surgical procedure. What can cause this to happen?

_____

_____

_____

_____

4. A surgical patient may be burned by a prep solution that has been warmed. What are two other reasons a prep solution should not be warmed?

_____

_____

_____

_____

5. In addition to chemical and thermal burns, a patient is at risk for other injuries during the surgical prep. Name and describe one.

_____

_____

_____

Internet Exercise

Using the Internet as a research tool, write a brief statement concerning the importance of patient safety in the operating room. What risk management tools have been formulated to prevent patient injuries?

_____

_____

_____

_____

_____

SKILL EVALUATION CHECKLIST Urinary Catheterization (Male or Female)

Student's Name: _____ Date: _____

Task: Student demonstrates the ability to perform urinary catheterization.

Equipment and Supplies:
► Sterile gloves
► Catheter supplies

Evaluation Directions: Check or circle the appropriate number to indicate the student's performance level, using the following rating scale.

3 = PROFICIENT. Can complete the task quickly and accurately without direction.
2 = PARTIALLY PROFICIENT. Can do most of the task. Needs assistance. Needs constant supervision.
1 = LIMITED. Can do a limited amount of the task. Must be told what to do. Needs extremely close supervision.
0 = UNSATISFACTORY. Can do a limited amount of the task. Must be told what to do. Needs extremely close supervision.

Task Checklist	Rating	Self-Assessment	Instructor Assessment
1. Assemble all equipment and supplies.	0 1 2 3		
2. Wash hands.	0 1 2 3		
3. Open catheter kit.	0 1 2 3		
4. Position and expose patient.	0 1 2 3		
5. Don sterile gloves, using proper technique.	0 1 2 3		
6. Organize supplies, using sterile technique.	0 1 2 3		
7. Apply sterile drapes that are supplied in the catheterization kit.	0 1 2 3		
8. Cleanse meatus using the proper technique.	0 1 2 3		
9. Lubricate tip of catheter.	0 1 2 3		
10. Invert catheter, and look for urine return.	0 1 2 3		
11. Inflate balloon.	0 1 2 3		
12. Secure catheter to patient's leg, if needed.	0 1 2 3		
13. Wash hands after procedure.	0 1 2 3		
Total Score			

SCORE   39–35 = A
34–30 = B
29–25 = C
24 = not passing

Comments:

_____
_____
_____

Chapter 12
Anesthesia

Key Terms

Write the definition for each term.

1. Amnesia: _____

_____

_____

2. Analgesia: _____

_____

_____

3. Anesthesia: _____

_____

_____

4. Anesthesia care provider (ACP): _____

_____

_____

5. Anesthesia machines: _____

_____

_____

6. Anesthesiologist: _____

_____

_____

7. Anesthetic: _____

_____

_____

8. Antagonist: _____

_____

_____

9. Anterograde amnesia: _____

_____

_____

10. Anxiolysis: _____

_____

_____

11. Apnea: _____

_____

_____

12. Bier block: _____

_____

_____

13. Bronchospasm: _____

_____

_____

14. Certified registered nurse anesthetist (CRNA): _____

_____

_____

15. Controlled hypothermia: _____

_____

_____

16. Cricoid pressure: _____

_____

_____

17. Delirium: _____

_____

_____

18. Drug: _____

_____

_____

19. Emergence: _____

_____

_____

20. Endotracheal tube: _____

_____

_____

21. Esmarch bandage: _____

_____

_____

22. Gas scavenging: _____

_____

_____

23. General anesthesia: _____

_____

_____

24. Homeostasis: _____

_____

_____

25. Induced hypotension: _____

_____

_____

26. Induction: _____

_____

_____

27. Intubation: _____

_____

_____

28. Laryngeal mask airway (LMA): _____

_____

_____

29. Laryngoscope: _____

_____

_____

30. Laryngospasm: _____

_____

_____

31. Malignant hyperthermia: _____

_____

_____

32. Medication: _____

_____

_____

33. Neuromuscular blocking agents: _____

_____

_____

34. Patent: _____

_____

_____

35. Pneumatic tourniquet: _____

_____

_____

36. Pulse oximeter: _____

_____

_____

37. Regional block: _____

_____

_____

38. Sedatives: _____

_____

_____

39. Synergistic: _____

_____

_____

40. Ventilation: _____

_____

_____

Short Answers

41. Who or what is an anesthesia care provider?

_____

_____

_____

_____

42. Monitoring the patient during surgery is a critical aspect of general anesthesia. Identify and briefly describe three ways in which the anesthesia care provider monitors the patient during surgery.

_____

_____

_____

_____

43. Describe sedation, analgesia, and amnesia.

_____

_____

_____

_____

44. Anesthesia induction is the passage from consciousness to unconsciousness. Explain how induction drugs are selected and how induction may be achieved.

_____

_____

_____

_____

45. After induction, the surgical level of anesthesia must be maintained throughout the operative procedure. Explain how the anesthesia care provider controls the patient's level of consciousness.

_____

_____

_____

_____

46. Describe a closed ventilation system.

_____

_____

_____

_____

47. As long as there is a patient in the room, suction must be available to the anesthesia care provider. Explain why this is important.

_____

_____

_____

_____

48. Thermal heating blankets are used by anesthesia personnel to help maintain the patient's core body temperature. Explain the risk to the patient if this device is faulty or improperly used.

_____

_____

_____

_____

49. Malignant hyperthermia is a rare event but can happen in the operating room. What is the scrubbed surgical technologist's role during a malignant hyperthermia crisis?

_____

_____

_____

_____

50. Describe the surgical technologist's role during a surgical patient's cardiac arrest.

_____

_____

_____

_____

Matching

Match each term with the correct definition. Some definitions will not be used.

A. ventilation

B. anterograde amnesia

C. cricoid pressure

D. laryngoscope

E. certified registered
   nurse anesthetist

F. general anesthesia

G. anesthesia

H. pulse oximeter

I. apnea

J. laryngospasm

K. anesthesiologist

L. intubation

M. bronchospasm

_____ 51. A physician who is a specialist in anesthesia and pain management

_____ 52. Movement of gases into and out of the lungs

_____ 53. A lighted instrument consisting of a blade and removable handle or a
       fiber optic light, used to assist in endotracheal intubation

_____ 54. A registered nurse trained and licensed to administer anesthetic agents

_____ 55. Cessation of breathing

_____ 56. An involuntary smooth muscle spasm of the bronchi

_____ 57. Compresses the trachea; helps prevent aspiration and can facilitate
       intubation

_____ 58. Involuntary smooth muscle spasms of the larynx

_____ 59. The process of inserting an endotracheal tube

_____ 60. Without sensation

True/False

Indicate whether the sentence or statement is true (T) or false (F).

_____ 61. It is critical for the surgical technologist to verify the amount of irrigation used during a surgical procedure and communicate this to the anesthesia care provider so he or she can accurately predict
blood loss.

_____ 62. All regional anesthetics are absorbed into the body, metabolized, and excreted.

_____ 63. The preoperative anesthesia history will not contain information about family history of complications during anesthesia.

_____ 64. All health-care workers should maintain current certification in cardiopulmonary resuscitation and
be able to respond in the event of cardiopulmonary arrest.

_____ 65. The anesthesia care provider is usually not the person directing resuscitation efforts.

_____ 66. All inhalation anesthetics, with the exception of nitrous oxide, are associated with malignant hyperthermia events.

_____ 67. Rocuronium or Zemuron is the only depolarizing muscle relaxant used in surgery.

_____ 68. Skeletal muscle relaxants are used in surgery as an adjunct to general anesthesia to permit tissue manipulation, especially during intubation.

_____ 69. Agents to reverse the effects of narcotic analgesics displace opiates from their receptor sites in the central nervous system and arrest their action. The most commonly used opiate reversal agent is naloxone or narcan.

_____ 70. Induced hypotension is the deliberate lowering of the patient's blood pressure to control hemorrhage and decrease the presence of blood at the surgical site.

Case Studies

Read the following case studies and answer the questions based on your knowledge of anesthesia in the surgical technology field.

Case 1: A healthy, 32-year-old female presents for bone marrow donation for transplantation. Her primary care physician contacts the anesthesiologist to report that the patient is extremely anxious about the procedure. The primary care physician requests that the anesthesiologist not discuss the risks associated with anesthesia in front of the patient, since it might "scare" her into not providing bone marrow for a sick aunt.

1. Do you think the anesthesiologist should honor the primary care physician's request? Why?

_____

_____

_____

_____

2. Do you think the anesthesia care provider may be able to reassure the patient by talking to her and explaining the anesthesia procedures?

_____

_____

_____

_____

3. If the anesthesiologist were to honor the primary care physician's request, would his or her decision be an unethical one? Explain your answer.

_____

_____

_____

_____

Case 2: The process for obtaining an informed consent for surgery usually begins before the patient enters the operating room environment, upon the patient's first visit to the surgeon's office. On the other hand, the informed consent for anesthesia is often obtained in the minutes before surgery, during which the anesthesiologist and patient meet for the first time.

1. What are some common situations in which a patient's ability to make decisions about surgery and anesthesia may be questioned?

_____

_____

_____

_____

2. What is done in an emergency, or when the patient is incapable of making a decision?

_____

_____

_____

_____

3. What if the patient requests not to hear about the risks associated with anesthesia and the surgery?

_____

_____

_____

_____

Internet Exercise

"Medical futility" refers to interventions that are unlikely to produce any significant benefit for the patient. Two kinds of medical futility are often distinguished. Using the Internet as a research tool, write a brief paragraph describing the two types of medical futility. Write a second paragraph describing what you feel the surgeon's ethical obligations are concerning a procedure that is deemed futile.

_____

_____

_____

_____

_____

_____

_____

_____

_____

_____

_____

_____

_____

_____

SKILL EVALUATION CHECKLIST Sellick's Maneuver

Student's Name: _____ Date: _____

Task: Student verbalizes purpose of cricoid pressure.

Equipment and Supplies:
▶ No equipment required

Evaluation Directions: Check or circle the appropriate number to indicate the student's performance level, using the following rating scale.

3 = PROFICIENT. Can complete the task quickly and accurately without direction.
2 = PARTIALLY PROFICIENT. Can do most of the task. Needs assistance. Needs constant supervision.
1 = LIMITED. Can do a limited amount of the task. Must be told what to do. Needs extremely close supervision.
0 = UNSATISFACTORY. Can do a limited amount of the task. Must be told what to do. Needs extremely close supervision.

Task Checklist	Rating	Self-Assessment	Instructor Assessment
1. Position self properly.	0 1 2 3		
2. Identify relevant anatomy.	0 1 2 3		
3. Position hand properly.	0 1 2 3		
4. Apply adequate pressure.	0 1 2 3		
5. Maintain cricoid pressure until asked to release.	0 1 2 3		
Total Score			

SCORE   39–35 = A
        34–30 = B
        29–25 = C
        24 = not passing

Comments:

_____

_____

_____

_____

Chapter 13
Surgical Pharmacology

Key Terms

Write the definition for each term.

1. Adverse reactions: _____

_____

_____

2. Antibiotic: _____

_____

_____

3. Anticoagulant: _____

_____

_____

4. Concentration: _____

_____

_____

5. Contrast medium: _____

_____

_____

6. Controlled substances: _____

_____

_____

7. Dosage: _____

_____

_____

8. Dose: _____

_____

_____

9. Drug: _____

_____

_____

10. Drug administration: _____

_____

_____

11. Dye: _____

_____

_____

12. Generic name: _____

_____

_____

13. Parenterally: _____

_____

_____

14. Pharmacodynamics: _____

_____

_____

15. Pharmacokinetics: _____

_____

_____

16. Pharmacology: _____

_____

_____

17. Prescription: _____

_____

_____

18. Side effects: _____

_____

_____

19. Stain: _____

_____

_____

20. Topical: _____

_____

_____

21. Trade name: _____

_____

_____

22. Transdermal: _____

_____

_____

23. U.S. Pharmacopeia (USP): _____

_____

_____

Short Answers

24. Before the surgical technologist passes any drug from the instrument table to the surgeon, he or she must do what?

   _____

   _____

   _____

   _____

25. Why must the surgical technologist be able to perform drug calculations?

   _____

   _____

   _____

   _____

26. There are standards for handling medications on the sterile field that should be strictly followed. These standards have been developed to protect patients and prevent medication errors. Briefly describe the procedure for accepting medication on the sterile field.

   _____

   _____

   _____

   _____

27. Measurement systems allow the quantification of physical properties. In medicine, the properties of concern are weight and volume. The two most commonly used measurement systems to specify these properties are the metric system and the apothecary system. Define each system.

   _____

   _____

   _____

   _____

28. What role does the Food and Drug Administration play in drug approval and standards?

_____

_____

_____

_____

29. Drugs that have potential for abuse are ranked based on the risk of abuse or dependency, harmful effects, and other factors. Lists of drugs with various rankings are called drug schedules. Who is responsible for determining the classification of drugs on these schedules? List the schedules, and give an example of a drug in each category.

_____

_____

_____

_____

30. Each drug has three names, generic, trade, and chemical. Only the generic and trade names are used in the health-care setting. Define generic name and trade name.

_____

_____

_____

_____

31. To help prevent medication errors, the five rights of medication errors were defined for administering medications in the health-care setting. A sixth right was added for surgical procedures. List these six rights.

_____

_____

_____

_____

_____

_____

_____

32. What is the responsibility of the surgical technologist in the scrub role regarding tracking the amount of drugs or solutions used during a surgical procedure?

_____

_____

_____

_____

33. Why are intravenous fluids given during surgery?

_____

_____

_____

Medication Calculations

34. Calculate a patient's weight by converting pounds to kilograms. Divide 2.2 into the number of pounds (2.2 kilograms = 1 pound).

   A. 125 lbs = _____ kg

   B. 60 lbs = _____ kg

   C. 200 lbs = _____ kg

   D. 150 lbs = _____ kg

   E. 30 lbs = _____ kg

   Carry your answers to the 100th (e.g., 5.33 kg).

35. Addition:

   A. 10cc of methylene blue added to 50cc of normal saline equals _____ ml?

   B. You have 5,000 units of heparin in lcc. The surgeon asks for 2,500 units of heparin in 25cc of normal saline. What is the total volume of solution? _____

   C. The surgeon's preference card states that he wants 50,000u of bacitracin mixed into 1,000cc of normal saline irrigation solution. Bacitracin 50,000u is packaged in a bottle in dry form and must be reconstituted prior to administration. Explain the procedure for mixing and receiving this medication on the sterile field.

   _____

   _____

   _____

   _____

Matching

Match each term with the correct definition.

A. pharmacokinetics

B. anticoagulant

C. dosage

D. pharmacodynamics

E. concentration

F. parenterally

G. dose

H. adverse reaction

I. transdermal

J. side effects

_____ 36. Refers to the administration of a drug through a skin patch impregnated with a drug

_____ 37. Anticipated effects of a drug other than those intended

_____ 38. Unexpected reactions to a drug that are not related to the dose

_____ 39. A drug that prolongs blood-clotting time

_____ 40. The movement of a drug through the tissues and cells of the body, including the process of absorption, distribution, and localization in tissues, biotransformation, and excretion by mechanical and chemical means

_____ 41. Refers to the administration of a drug by injection

_____ 42. The quantity of a drug to be taken at one time, or the stated amount of drug per unit of distribution

_____ 43. The regulated administration of prescribed amounts of a drug

_____ 44. The biochemical and physiologic effects of drugs and their mechanisms of action in the body

_____ 45. A measure of the quantity of a substance per a specific volume or weight

True/False

Indicate whether the sentence or statement is true (T) or false (F).

_____ 46. Drug action is in part regulated by the route of administration. Serious drug errors and death can result from the wrong route delivery of drugs.

_____ 47. Petrolatum gauze and other types of sticky material should be grasped with forceps to remove them from the wrappers; the oils in these products may weaken surgical gloves.

_____ 48. When measuring drugs in a syringe or other measuring device, you must read the value at the top of the curve formed by the liquid in a container.

_____ 49. When relieving another surgical technologist in the scrub role, you find that he or she has not labeled the drugs on the sterile field. You should discard them and have the correct drugs redistributed to the field and properly label them immediately.

_____ 50. When passing a drug to the surgeon, it is the surgical technologist's responsibility to announce the name and concentration of the drug.

_____ 51. The surgical technologist in the scrub role may insert a needle into a vial held by the circulator to obtain drugs. If done properly, this will not put the circulator at risk for a needle stick.

_____ 52. A number of drugs are manufactured as powders and mixed with a sterile diluent. It is acceptable to use more diluent but never less than specified by the surgeon's orders.

_____ 53. Never use an insulin syringe to measure drugs on the sterile field.

_____ 54. Never recap a needle by hand. Place the cap on a flat surface, and scoop it up with the point of the needle.

_____ 55. It is not necessary to label irrigating saline or sterile water on the back table.

Case Study

Read the following case study and answer the questions based on your knowledge of surgical pharmacology in the surgical technology field.

The surgical setting differs from other settings. Many medication orders are given verbally or originate from a surgeon's preference card. Moving medications to the sterile field may result in having multiple unlabeled medications available. High-alert medications, including the "caines" and epinephrine, are available in multiple dosage forms and concentrations.

1. There are standards for handling and accepting medications on the sterile field. Write a short paragraph describing the standards developed to protect the patient and to prevent medication errors in the surgical setting.

   _____

   _____

   _____

   _____

2. What makes the surgical setting different from other settings in the health-care facility where patients may receive medications?

   _____

   _____

   _____

   _____

3. Why is labeling medications on the sterile field important?

   _____

   _____

   _____

   _____

4. What should the labels contain?

_____

_____

_____

_____

5. Should the surgical technologist label sterile water and NaCl on the sterile field?

_____

_____

_____

_____

Internet Exercises

1. Research the history of pharmacology. How were some common medications discovered?

_____

_____

2. Use the Internet to look up information for your drug cards.

3. Look up the U.S. Metric Association.

SKILL EVALUATION CHECKLIST: Draw Up Medication in a Syringe into the Sterile Field

Student's Name: _____ Date: _____

Task: Student identifies proper medication and accepts medication onto sterile field.

Equipment and Supplies:
▶ Proper medication
▶ Alcohol prep
▶ Appropriate syringe and needle

Evaluation Directions: Check or circle the appropriate number to indicate the student's performance level, using the following rating scale.

3 = PROFICIENT. Can complete the task quickly and accurately without direction.
2 = PARTIALLY PROFICIENT. Can do most of the task. Needs assistance. Needs constant supervision.
1 = LIMITED. Can do a limited amount of the task. Must be told what to do. Needs extremely close supervision.
0 = UNSATISFACTORY. Can do a limited amount of the task. Must be told what to do. Needs extremely close supervision.

Task Checklist	Rating	Self-Assessment	Instructor Assessment
1. Verify patient allergies.	0 1 2 3		
2. Circulator prepares medication for withdrawal.	0 1 2 3		
3. STSR and circulator visually and verbally confirm correct medication.	0 1 2 3		
4. STSR withdraws medication from container using proper technique.	0 1 2 3		
5. STSR and circulator visually and verbally confirm correct medication.	0 1 2 3		
6. Medication is labeled on the field.	0 1 2 3		
7. Medication is passed to surgeon when requested and verbally identified.	0 1 2 3		
Total Score			

SCORE   39–35 = A
        34–30 = B
        29–25 = C
        24 = not passing

Comments:

_____

_____

_____

_____

Chapter 14
Environmental Hazards

Key Terms

Write the definition for each term.

1. Airborne transmission precautions: _____

    _____

    _____

2. Blood-borne pathogens: _____

    _____

    _____

3. Genetic mutation: _____

    _____

    _____

4. Latex: _____

    _____

    _____

5. Needleless system: _____

    _____

    _____

6. Neutral zone (no-hands) technique: _____

    _____

    _____

7. Occupational exposure: _____

_____

_____

8. Personal protective equipment: _____

_____

_____

9. Postexposure prophylaxis: _____

_____

_____

10. Potentially infectious materials: _____

_____

_____

11. Risk: _____

_____

_____

12. Sharps: _____

_____

_____

13. Smoke plume: _____

_____

_____

14. Standard precautions: _____

_____

_____

15. Transmission-based precautions: _____

_____

_____

Short Answers

16. What risk factors place surgical personnel at high risk for occupational and environmental injuries?

_____

_____

_____

_____

17. The risk of fire is greater in the operating room than in other health-care settings. List three causes of fire in the operating room.

_____

_____

_____

_____

18. List the fuel sources for fire at the operative site.

_____

_____

_____

_____

19. Health-care workers are at high risk of exposure to diseases spread by airborne particles, aerosol droplets, blood, and other body fluids. To minimize the risk to workers and patients, OSHA and the CDC have developed a set of recommendations and precautions. Define standard precautions.

_____

_____

_____

_____

20. Although the nature of blood-borne disease and its transmission and prevention methods are known to health-care workers, the human factor must be included in the planning and implementation of any risk-reduction program. Identify several reasons health-care workers have difficulty in risk reduction.

_____

_____

_____

_____

21. Smoke plume contains a number of toxic chemicals in concentrations that can potentially exceed those recommended by OSHA. The potential hazards of these substances are infectious disease transmission, toxicity from chemicals, and allergy. What is smoke plume?

_____

_____

_____

_____

22. Sensitivity and a true allergy to latex rubber are a risk to both patients and personnel in health care. Define and describe a latex allergy.

_____

_____

_____

_____

23. Although lead aprons are uncomfortable and heavy, surgical team members should wear them under their sterile surgical gowns during any procedure that requires radiation. Identify the risks of repeated exposure or overexposure to radiation.

_____

_____

_____

_____

24. Operating room personnel are exposed to many different types of chemicals. Many of these are hazardous and can produce serious long-term effects such as respiratory or skin problems. List several chemicals that a surgical technologist will be exposed to in the operating room.

_____

_____

_____

_____

25. Musculoskeletal injury is a risk for all personnel working in the operating room. Identify three causes of musculoskeletal injury in the operating room.

_____

_____

_____

_____

Matching

Match each term with the correct definition.

A. latex

B. occupational exposure

C. neutral zone

D. smoke plume

E. risk

F. standard precautions

G. transmission-based precautions

H. postexposure prophylaxis

I. blood-borne pathogens

J. "RACE"

_____ 26. A plan based on four immediate actions to be taken by health-care personnel to protect patients and staff in the event of a fire

_____ 27. A naturally occurring sap obtained from rubber trees and used in the manufacture of medical devices and other commercial goods

_____ 28. A method of transferring sharp instruments on the surgical field without hand-to-hand contact

_____ 29. Standards and precautions to prevent the spread of infectious diseases by patients known to be infected

_____ 30. Recommended procedures to help prevent the development of blood-borne diseases after an exposure incident

_____ 31. The statistical probability of a given event based on the number of such events that have already occurred in a certain population

_____ 32. Examples are the hepatitis B virus and the human immunodeficiency virus

_____ 33. Exposure to hazards in the workplace

_____ 34. Contains toxic chemicals, vapors, blood fragments, and viruses

_____ 35. Standards and procedures to prevent the transmission of infectious diseases

True/False

Indicate whether the sentence or statement is true (T) or false (F).

_____ 36. Dosimeters are available to measure the cumulative radiation dose for those who are frequently exposed to radiation.

_____ 37. When lifting an object, hold it as far from your body as possible. This decreases the force of exertion.

_____ 38. Toxic chemicals can only enter the body through skin that is not intact.

_____ 39. Failure to check a patient's latex allergy before surgery can lead to serious injury or death.

_____ 40. Both laser and electrosurgical smoke plumes contain living and dead cells.

_____ 41. Waste bags for infectious material are red.

_____ 42. It is not necessary to wear gloves when handling certain tissue specimens.

_____ 43. Monopolar devices do not require the use of a grounding pad (dispersive electrodes).

_____ 44. The most frequent source of electrical injury to the surgical patient is from the electrosurgical unit (ESU).

_____ 45. If an electrical instrument begins to malfunction during surgery, it must be sent to biomedical engineering if the surgical technologist cannot get it to work properly.

Case Studies

Read the following case studies and answer the questions based on your knowledge of environmental hazards in the surgical technology field.

Case 1: A 63-year-old male patient underwent a transurethral resection of the prostate that took approximately 45 minutes to complete. An electrosurgical unit (ESU) was used for the procedure. The anesthesia provider connected an ECG monitor to the patient. The circulating nurse set up the ESU, and the dial was initially set at three in the cut mode. The dial setting was increased from three to seven at the surgeon's request. Before his request for the setting to be increased, a member of the OR staff tripped on the dispersive electrode cable. The dispersive electrode was applied to the lateral left thigh before the patient was placed in the lithotomy position for the procedure. The electrode was not checked for proper contact with the patient following repositioning. After the procedure, as the drapes were being removed from the patient, it was noted that the conductive portion of the dispersive electrode was no longer in contact with the patient. There was no injury beneath the dispersive electrode. However, a routine postoperative skin check revealed an area of skin injury behind the patient's knee, which had been in contact with a portion of the metal knee support. The knee supports were covered with padding, except where a portion had been worn away. The injured area was a light cream color, was hard to the touch, and had a red rim. It measured approximately 2 × 3.5 cm.

1. What caused the patient's injury?

_____

_____

_____

_____

2. What precautions should have been taken to avoid the patient's injury?

_____

_____

_____

_____

Case 2: Dana is the surgical technologist for a mini-laparotomy for a tubal ligation procedure. She places the scalpel in a basin. When Dr. Keller, the surgeon, asks for the scalpel, she hands him the basin. He asks, "What is this?" How should Dana respond?

_____

_____

_____

_____

Internet Exercise

Some hospitals sort trash into noncontaminated (plastic), noncontaminated ("other"), and contaminated (red bag) trash. Using the Internet as a research tool, write a brief paragraph on how medical facilities dispose of medical waste contained in red biohazard bags.

_____

_____

_____

_____

_____

_____

Chapter 15
Surgical Techniques

Key Terms

Write the definition for each term.

1. Biopsy: _____

   _____

2. Bleeder: _____

   _____

3. Blunt dissection: _____

   _____

4. Case planning: _____

   _____

5. Count: _____

   _____

6. Culture: _____

   _____

7. Eschar: _____

   _____

8. Frozen section: _____

   _____

9. Implant: _____

   _____

10. Sharp dissection: _____

_____

11. Sharps: _____

_____

12. Stent dressing: _____

_____

Short Answers

13. Surgical procedures can be classified into five categories. A knowledge of these categories can aid in planning cases, because surgical procedures in a specific category require common skills and techniques. Identify the five categories, and briefly describe each.

_____

_____

_____

_____

14. Prior to opening sterile supplies for a case, list the steps that should be taken by the surgical technologist to ensure that all needed equipment is available and working properly.

_____

_____

_____

_____

15. When opening sterile supplies for a surgical case, they are opened in a logical manner. What should be opened first? Why?

_____

_____

_____

_____

16. Why is it important to use a methodical approach with all setups?

_____

_____

_____

_____

17. It is important to know and understand the preliminary steps of a procedure in order. This concept is very important during an emergency procedure when there is no time to organize equipment before the patient is brought into the room. List five steps in sequence that will allow you to have the "priority" equipment ready that is needed to start the case.

_____

_____

_____

_____

18. List the different types of surgical sponges and the uses for each.

_____

_____

_____

_____

19. Policies directing sponge, sharps, and instrument counts have been established by the Joint Commission for the Accreditation of Healthcare Organizations, the Association of periOperative Nurses, and the Association of Surgical Technologists. Hospitals create their own policies based on those of the accrediting and professional organizations. Explain why surgical counts are performed.

_____

_____

_____

_____

20. You are the surgical technologist in the scrub role on an exploratory laparotomy. The frozen section was positive for carcinoma. The surgery was more extensive than planned, and there was more blood loss than expected. There is a shift change, and you are being relieved by another scrub. A sponge (RAYTEC) is missing and a lap sponge is missing. What will you do?

_____

_____

_____

_____

21. Surgical instruments are the domain of the surgical technologist. Discuss the special properties of instruments and the need for care when passing instruments to the surgeon.

_____

_____

_____

_____

22. Discuss the neutral zone or "no-hands" technique.

_____

_____

_____

_____

23. During surgery, tissue is often removed for pathologic analysis. Critical medical decisions are made based on specimen analysis. Each person who handles a specimen has a responsibility for its protection, preservation, and identification. Explain the consequences of the improper handling of specimens.

_____

_____

_____

_____

24. Discuss why the unnecessary and rough handling of tissue can be detrimental to a surgical patient. List the steps that can be taken to prevent this from happening.

_____

_____

_____

_____

25. List and discuss wound drainage. What are the two methods? List and give examples of each method, listing the specific drain and where or why it would be used.

_____

_____

_____

_____

Matching

Match each term with the correct definition.

A. culture

B. frozen section

C. stent dressing

D. biopsy

E. eschar

F. sharp dissection

G. blunt dissection

H. implant

I. kick bucket

J. nonadherent barrier

_____ 26. Gauze strips or squares impregnated with plain or antibacterial ointment, used for dressings where dressing changes must not cause disruption of tissue healing or bleeding

_____ 27. Used laparotomy and 4 × 4 sponges are dropped into this receptacle by the surgical technologist in the scrub role for retrieval by the circulator to be isolated for counts

_____ 28. A process in which a sample of exudates, pus, or fluid is grown in culture media and analyzed for the presence of infectious microorganisms

_____ 29. Removal of a sample of tissue for pathologic analysis

_____ 30. The technique of cutting tissue using instruments such as a knife, scissors, or an electrosurgical tip

_____ 31. Tissue that is burned to the point of carbonization

_____ 32. A thin slice of tissue obtained during surgery for immediate analysis

_____ 33. A synthetic or metal replacement for an anatomical structure such as a joint or cranial bone

_____ 34. The technique of separating tissue layers by teasing them apart with a sponge dissector

_____ 35. Any type of dressing in which a molded pressure dressing is sutured to the wound site

True/False

Indicate whether the sentence or statement is true (T) or false (F).

———— 36. Some wounds require frequent dressing changes. Montgomery straps are a common type of abdominal binder used for these types of wounds.

———— 37. Packing is a method of filling a wound site or cavity with gauze material to absorb draining fluids or to purposely debride during the dressing change. The wound is sutured after each dressing change.

———— 38. A pressure dressing is the most commonly used dressing over a skin graft.

———— 39. Benzoin is commonly used on small superficial wounds to enhance the sticking ability of steri-strips.

———— 40. Only some dressings protect the wound from environmental contamination, but all provide pressure, support, skin closure, absorption, and debridement.

———— 41. When any drainage system is in use, the collection unit must remain at or above the level of the insertion tube.

———— 42. A drain is a device used to provide continuous or intermittent removal of serous fluid from a healing wound.

———— 43. The pneumatic tourniquet is a surgical device used to control venous and arterial circulation to create a bloodless surgical site during surgical procedures of limbs.

———— 44. The harmonic scalpel works much the same way that an electrosurgical unit works, using heat and producing eschar.

———— 45. Maintaining the body's total blood volume and controlling bleeding is called hemostasis.

Case Studies

Read the following case studies and answer the questions based on your knowledge of surgical technique in the surgical technology field.

Case 1: A 72-year-old female underwent right aortoiliac aneurysm repair. She developed postoperative fever, initially attributed to ventilator-associated pneumonia. However, the fever persisted, and no definite source was identified. The patient received multiple courses of broad-spectrum antibiotics over a 2-month hospital stay. Several months after discharge, she was admitted to another facility with recurrent fever, neurological deficits, and renal failure. The patient was diagnosed as having endocarditis with *Candida albicans* based on echocardiography and blood culture results. Despite amphotericin B and valve surgery, she died a few weeks after this admission. Autopsy revealed a surgical sponge in the abdomen around the previous aortoiliac repair. An abdominal computed tomography (CT) scan during the stay in the previous hospital had shown a metal clip in the area of the graft, but no other abnormalities. The patient had not undergone any other surgical procedures.

1. What could have been the cause of this patient's death?

_____

_____

_____

_____

2. What could have prevented the sponge from being left in the surgical wound?

_____

_____

_____

_____

3. If the surgical counts had been performed and the count was incorrect, what steps could have been taken to retrieve the lost sponge?

_____

_____

_____

_____

4. The loss of sponges, needles, instruments, and other equipment not only poses a serious risk to the patient, it also creates other problems. List additional problems caused by lost and retained items.

_____

_____

_____

_____

5. When should a count be performed?

_____

_____

_____

_____

Case 2: Elizabeth, a 63-year-old female, has been admitted to the emergency department with severe abdominal pain after a motor vehicle crash. She is being brought to the operating room for an emergency laparotomy.

1. What should the surgical technologist's concern be as he or she begins to set up for this case?

   _____

   _____

   _____

   _____

2. What should the preliminary steps be for this procedure?

   _____

   _____

   _____

   _____

3. Which items would be critical to have ready during an emergency procedure such as this?

   _____

   _____

   _____

   _____

4. Why is it important to know and understand the steps of a surgical procedure?

   _____

   _____

   _____

   _____

5. Describe some duties of the surgical technologist during this case.

   _____

   _____

   _____

   _____

Internet Exercise

Any nontissue item removed from the surgical patient is considered a specimen. Some specimens such as bullets and knife blades are forensic evidence and used for legal purposes. All hospitals should have policies and procedures that outline traumatic injuries and death, staff responsibilities, and details of collecting evidence, documentation, and chain of custody. The procedure also should include care of victims, suspected perpetrators, and the family or persons accompanying the patient. Using the Internet as a research tool, write a brief paragraph on the protocol that may be used for forensic or legal evidence obtained in the surgical setting.

_____

_____

_____

_____

_____

_____

Chapter 16
Sutures and Wound Healing

Key Terms

Write the definition for each term.

1. Absorbable sutures: _____

   _____

   _____

2. Anastomosis: _____

   _____

   _____

3. Approximate: _____

   _____

   _____

4. Bleeder: _____

   _____

   _____

5. Blunt needle: _____

   _____

   _____

6. Bolsters: _____

   _____

   _____

7. Brown and Sharp (B & S) gauge: _____

_____

_____

8. Capillarity: _____

_____

_____

9. Chromic salt: _____

_____

_____

10. Control-release: _____

_____

_____

11. Dehiscence: _____

_____

_____

12. Double-armed sutures: _____

_____

_____

13. Elasticity: _____

_____

_____

14. Evisceration: _____

_____

_____

15. First intention wound closure: _____

_____

_____

16. Inert: _____

_____

_____

17. Interrupted suture: _____

_____

_____

18. Keith needle: _____

_____

_____

19. Ligate: _____

_____

_____

20. Ligature: _____

_____

_____

21. Mattress suture: _____

_____

_____

22. Memory: _____

_____

_____

23. Monofilament suture: _____

_____

_____

24. Multifilament suture: _____

_____

_____

25. Nonabsorbable sutures: _____

_____

_____

26. Pliability: _____

_____

_____

27. Purse-string: _____

_____

_____

28. Reel: _____

_____

_____

29. Retention suture: _____

_____

_____

30. Reverse cutting needles: _____

_____

_____

31. Running suture: _____

_____

_____

32. Second intention wound closure: _____

_____

_____

33. Stick tie: _____

_____

_____

34. Swaged needle: _____

_____

_____

35. Tensile strength: _____

_____

_____

36. Third intention wound closure: _____

_____

_____

37. Throw: _____

_____

_____

38. Tie-down: _____

_____

_____

39. Tie on a passer: _____

_____

_____

40. Tissue drag: _____

_____

_____

Short Answers

41. What are suture materials used for?

_____

_____

_____

_____

42. All substances, including suture products that bear the USP label, must meet minimum standards. Standards for suture materials include what?

_____

_____

_____

_____

43. When selecting sutures for a case, always check the expiration date. Why should sutures whose date has expired not be used?

_____

_____

_____

_____

44. What are the desired qualities for selecting sutures?

_____

_____

_____

_____

45. Suture material is foreign to the body; the body recognizes it as "nonself." The body's immune system reacts to sutures as it would to any foreign material. The tissue becomes inflamed, and the body attempts to destroy the foreign material by breaking down the sutures. High reactivity to sutures causes what?

_____

_____

_____

_____

46. List four configurations of sutures and the design of each stand.

_____

_____

_____

_____

47. The following terms commonly apply to sutures: absorbable, nonabsorbable, synthetic, natural. Define each term, and list a suture that applies to each.

_____

_____

_____

_____

48. Surgical needles have three distinct parts. Identify each part.

_____

_____

_____

_____

49. Identify and describe the type of suture used to approximate blood vessels or other tubular structures.

_____

_____

_____

_____

50. Wound healing is described by the technique used to close the wound. Define first intention, second intention, and third intention.

_____

_____

_____

Matching

Match each term with the correct definition.

A. dehiscence

B. capillarity

C. tensile strength

D. tissue drag

E. pliability

F. memory

G. evisceration

H. anastomosis

I. Brown and Sharp (B & S) gauge

J. Inert

_____ 51. The separation of the layers of the surgical wound, which may be partial and superficial only, or a complete disruption of all layers

_____ 52. To create a connection between two vessels or two normally separated spaces or organs

_____ 53. The quality that produces friction between the suture and the tissue

_____ 54. The flexibility of a suture

_____ 55. The amount of force or stress a suture can withstand without breaking. This term also is used to refer to the strength of tissues as they heal

_____ 56. Sizing standard used to measure the diameter of wire or stainless steel

_____ 57. The protrusion of abdominal contents through a wound or through a surgical incision that has failed

_____ 58. The ability of suture material to soak up fluid along the strand from the immersed, wet end into the dry, nonimmersed end

_____ 59. For suture material, the recoil of the suture after it has been removed from the package

_____ 60. Sutures and implants that because of their biochemical properties provoke little or no inflammatory reaction in the body

True/False

Indicate whether the sentence or statement is true (T) or false (F).

_____ 61. A hematoma or blood-filled pocket may become a reservoir for infection.

_____ 62. Nutrition is not considered an important contribution to rapid wound healing.

_____ 63. To prevent wound dehiscence, retention sutures are commonly placed to reinforce primary suture lines.

_____ 64. Areas that do not heal quickly are those that are vascular, including the head, face, mouth, and mucous membranes.

_____ 65. Wound healing occurs in one stage.

_____ 66. The primary use of a tissue adhesive is to seal the bleeding surface of a vascular organ, such as the liver, spleen, or intestine.

_____ 67. When using surgical staplers, tissue handling becomes more frequent, thus increasing trauma by manipulation and exposure.

_____ 68. When passing clip appliers, pass with the tip down, taking care not to squeeze the handles and releasing the clip prematurely.

_____ 69. The needle holder is passed to the surgeon with the point of the needle aimed toward his or her chin.

_____ 70. The positioning of the needle holder in relation to the suture needle depends on whether the surgical technologist is left-handed or right-handed.

Case Studies

Read the following case studies and answer the questions based on your knowledge of sutures and wound healing in the surgical technology field.

Case 1: Joan, a 53-year-old female, has been suffering from right-upper-quadrant pain. She has been admitted to the emergency department for diagnostic studies. The results of her studies confirm the presence of gallstones. Her surgeon has scheduled Joan for an open cholecystectomy with a common bile duct exploration. Joan is a noncompliant diabetic and morbidly obese.

1. What is the expected surgical wound classification of Joan's procedure?

   _____

   _____

   _____

   _____

2. By which method will Joan's wound be expected to heal?

   _____

   _____

   _____

   _____

3. Given Joan's underlying conditions, what considerations should be made during closure of the surgical wound?

_____

_____

_____

_____

4. Explain the possible complications of wound healing for which Joan may be at risk.

_____

_____

_____

_____

5. List two factors that will influence Joan's surgical wound healing time.

_____

_____

_____

_____

Case 2: You are the surgical technologist; the surgeon is working deep in the abdomen of an obese patient, and suddenly he asks you for a tie. What will you pass to him, and how will you pass it?

_____

_____

_____

_____

Internet Exercise

Wound closure techniques have evolved from the earliest development of suturing materials to comprise resources that include synthetic sutures, absorbable sutures, staples, tapes, and adhesive compounds. The engineering of sutures in synthetic material, along with the standardization of traditional materials (e.g., catgut, silk), has produced superior aesthetic results. Similarly, the creation of natural glues, surgical staples, and tapes to substitute for sutures has supplemented the choices available to surgeons today. Using the Internet as a research tool, write a brief paragraph on the use of tissue adhesive compounds in surgical procedures.

_____

_____

_____

_____

_____

_____

_____

SKILL EVALUATION CHECKLIST: Instrument Handling—Load, Pass, and Unload a Scalpel Handle

Student's Name: _____ Date: _____

Task: Student demonstrates knowledge of utilizing neutral zone when passing scalpels.

Equipment and Supplies:
▶ Scalpel blade
▶ Knife handle
▶ Needle driver
▶ Sharps container

Evaluation Directions: Check or circle the appropriate number to indicate the student's performance level, using the following rating scale.

3 = PROFICIENT. Can complete the task quickly and accurately without direction.
2 = PARTIALLY PROFICIENT. Can do most of the task. Needs assistance. Needs constant supervision.
1 = LIMITED. Can do a limited amount of the task. Must be told what to do. Needs extremely close supervision.
0 = UNSATISFACTORY. Can do a limited amount of the task. Must be told what to do. Needs extremely close supervision.

Task Checklist	Rating	Self-Assessment	Instructor Assessment
1. Scalpel blade is secured using needle driver.	0 1 2 3		
2. Blade is applied to handle using needle driver.	0 1 2 3		
3. Scalpel is placed in a designated neutral zone.	0 1 2 3		
4. Scalpel is retrieved from neutral zone.	0 1 2 3		
5. Blade is removed from handle using a needle driver.	0 1 2 3		
6. Dispose of blade properly.	0 1 2 3		
Total Score			

SCORE   39–35 = A
         34–30 = B
         29–25 = C
         24 = not passing

Comments:

_____

_____

_____

_____

SKILL EVALUATION CHECKLIST: Suture/Needle/Staple Handling—Load, Pass, and Unload a Needle Holder Using the Neutral Zone Technique

Student's Name: _____ Date: _____

Task: Student demonstrates knowledge of utilizing neutral zone when passing loaded needle drivers.

Equipment and Supplies:
▶ Proper suture
▶ Appropriate needle driver
▶ Appropriate additional instruments (forceps, scissors)
▶ Magnetic needle box

Evaluation Directions: Check or circle the appropriate number to indicate the student's performance level, using the following rating scale.

3 = PROFICIENT. Can complete the task quickly and accurately without direction.
2 = PARTIALLY PROFICIENT. Can do most of the task. Needs assistance. Needs constant supervision.
1 = LIMITED. Can do a limited amount of the task. Must be told what to do. Needs extremely close supervision.
0 = UNSATISFACTORY. Can do a limited amount of the task. Must be told what to do. Needs extremely close supervision.

Task Checklist	Rating	Self-Assessment	Instructor Assessment
1. Open suture packet.	0 1 2 3		
2. Needle driver is loaded using "no-touch" technique.	0 1 2 3		
3. Loaded needle driver is placed in the neutral zone.	0 1 2 3		
4. Appropriate instrument (forceps or scissors) is passed to surgeon.	0 1 2 3		
5. Needle driver is retrieved from the neutral zone.	0 1 2 3		
6. Suture needle is placed in magnetic needle box.	0 1 2 3		
Total Score			

SCORE   39–35 = A
            34–30 = B
            29–25 = C
            24 = not passing

Comments:

_____

_____

_____

SKILL EVALUATION CHECKLIST: Suture/Needle/Staple Handling—Load, Pass, and Unload a Needle Holder Using the Direct Passing Technique

Student's Name: _____ Date: _____

Task: Student demonstrates the ability to properly load suture material and safely pass suture to surgeon.

Equipment and Supplies:
▶ Proper suture
▶ Appropriate needle holder
▶ Appropriate additional instruments (forceps, scissors, or both)

Evaluation Directions: Check or circle the appropriate number to indicate the student's performance level, using the following rating scale.

3 = PROFICIENT. Can complete the task quickly and accurately without direction.
2 = PARTIALLY PROFICIENT. Can do most of the task. Needs assistance. Needs constant supervision.
1 = LIMITED. Can do a limited amount of the task. Must be told what to do. Needs extremely close supervision.
0 = UNSATISFACTORY. Can do a limited amount of the task. Must be told what to do. Needs extremely close supervision.

Task Checklist	Rating	Self-Assessment	Instructor Assessment
1. Open suture packet.	0 1 2 3		
2. Needle holder is loaded for right-handed or left-handed surgeon.	0 1 2 3		
3. Pass suture to surgeon.	0 1 2 3		
4. Pass additional instruments (forceps, Mayo scissors, or both).	0 1 2 3		
5. Suture needle is returned from field.	0 1 2 3		
6. Needle holder is reloaded or returned to proper place.	0 1 2 3		
Total Score			

SCORE   39–35 = A
            34–30 = B
            29–25 = C
            24 = not passing

Comments:

_____

_____

_____

_____

SKILL EVALUATION CHECKLIST: Suture/Needle/Staple Handling—Pass Ties (includes reel, free ties, and ties on a pass)

Student's Name: _____ Date: _____

Task: Student demonstrates knowledge of passing sutures for ties.

Equipment and Supplies:
▶ Suture material of various types
▶ Scissors
▶ Passer instrument (Mixter, hemostat)

Evaluation Directions: Check or circle the appropriate number to indicate the student's performance level, using the following rating scale.

3 = PROFICIENT. Can complete the task quickly and accurately without direction.
2 = PARTIALLY PROFICIENT. Can do most of the task. Needs assistance. Needs constant supervision.
1 = LIMITED. Can do a limited amount of the task. Must be told what to do. Needs extremely close supervision.
0 = UNSATISFACTORY. Can do a limited amount of the task. Must be told what to do. Needs extremely close supervision.

Task Checklist	Rating	Self-Assessment	Instructor Assessment
1. Select necessary suture.	0 1 2 3		
2. Prepare and pass a free tie.	0 1 2 3		
3. Prepare and pass tie on a passer.	0 1 2 3		
4. Pass scissors.	0 1 2 3		
Total Score			

SCORE 39–35 = A
34–30 = B
29–25 = C
24 = not passing

Comments:

_____

_____

_____

_____

Chapter 17
Laser Surgery and Electrosurgery

Key Terms

Write the definition for each term.

1. Ablation: _____

_____

_____

2. Active electrode: _____

_____

_____

3. Alternate site burn: _____

_____

_____

4. Ampere: _____

_____

_____

5. Amplification system: _____

_____

_____

6. Amplitude: _____

_____

_____

7. Circuit: _____

_____

_____

8. Coagulation: _____

_____

_____

9. Coherent: _____

_____

_____

10. Current: _____

_____

_____

11. Dispersive electrode: _____

_____

_____

12. Electromagnetic spectrum: _____

_____

_____

13. Frequency: _____

_____

_____

14. Fulguration: _____

_____

_____

15. Gas: _____

_____

_____

16. Infrared: _____

_____

_____

17. Laser: _____

_____

_____

18. Laser medium: _____

_____

_____

19. Laser safety officer: _____

_____

_____

20. Monochromatic: _____

_____

_____

21. Optical resonant cavity: _____

_____

_____

22. Parallel: _____

_____

_____

23. Photon: _____

_____

_____

24. Power: _____

_____

25. Pulsed wave: _____

_____

_____

26. Radiant exposure: _____

_____

_____

27. Semiconductor: _____

_____

_____

28. Solid: _____

_____

_____

29. Solid-state: _____

_____

_____

30. Voltage: _____

_____

_____

31. Wavelength: _____

_____

_____

Short Answers

32. Laser is an acronym for what?

_____

_____

_____

_____

33. Laser surgery is designed to cut or destroy diseased tissue without harming healthy, normal tissue. It also is designed to do what?

_____

_____

_____

_____

34. The laser is a powerful tool that has a variety of applications in manufacturing, engineering, biotechnology, health, and warfare. Laser technology has created a new field in medicine. However, lasers also have the capacity to cause what?

_____

_____

_____

_____

35. Explain what happens when a laser beam touches tissue.

_____

_____

_____

_____

36. The distinctive characteristics of laser energy are created when what occurs?

_____

_____

_____

_____

37. What are the effects caused by laser light on a surface?

_____

_____

_____

_____

38. The quality of laser energy differs depending on its density, which is determined by what?

_____

_____

_____

_____

39. Radiant exposure is the sum of what factors?

_____

_____

_____

_____

40. The argon gas laser produces a visible blue-green beam that is color specific and absorbed by brown-pigmented tissue such as hemoglobin. The argon laser is used most commonly in which procedures?

_____

_____

_____

_____

41. The carbon dioxide laser medium is a combination of helium, nitrogen, and carbon dioxide, and the beam is invisible to the human eye. The carbon dioxide laser has a high affinity for water and is used in which types of procedures?

_____

_____

_____

_____

Matching

Match each term with the correct definition.

A. laser safety officer

B. ablation

C. fulguration

D. radiant exposure

E. active electrode

F. circuit

G. dispersive electrode

H. coagulation

I. carbonization

J. alternate site burn

_____ 42. The closed path where current flows

_____ 43. Removal and destruction of tissue by erosion or vaporization, usually due to intense heat

_____ 44. Same as a fourth-degree burn; it occurs when the temperature of the electrode tip exceeds 200° C

_____ 45. A person who is knowledgeable in laser safety and use, assigned by the hospital to monitor and maintain safety standards for laser use

_____ 46. The total effect of laser energy, which depends on the energy density of the laser beam, the diameter of the beam, and the exposure time

_____ 47. An instrument or a device used in surgery to deliver concentrated electrical current to tissue

_____ 48. High-voltage superficial tissue coagulation; the electrode does not touch the tissue; also called spray coagulation

_____ 49. Clotting of blood

_____ 50. The grounding pad applied to the patient that directs current flow from the patient back to the power unit

_____ 51. A patient burn at a site other than the target tissue, which has many causes

True/False

Indicate whether the sentence or statement is true (T) or false (F).

_____ 52. Remove tissue and eschar from the active electrode tip with a knife blade or other sharp instrument.

_____ 53. Electrosurgery carries a high risk of patient and environmental fire, especially in the presence of flammable preparation solutions. If these solutions must be used, make sure that the skin is completely dry before draping the patient.

_____ 54. Impedance is probably the least well understood concept in electrosurgery. It refers to the flow of electrical current into structures that are not designed to be a part of the electrical current.

_____ 55. Tissues with a high liquid content are more resistant to the flow of electricity than tissues with less water content.

_____ 56. Increasing the voltage of the ESU beyond normal levels without investigating why a higher voltage is needed would not result in a severe injury to the patient.

_____ 57. The dispersive electrode pad should be placed in a fleshy area with uniform contact to the skin. The pad should not be placed over a bony protuberance but over a highly vascularized area.

_____ 58. A dispersive electrode is not required with the use of a bipolar unit.

_____ 59. It is not the surgical technologist's responsibility to know and understand the use of electrosurgical equipment in the surgical setting; it is the circulator's responsibility.

_____ 60. When using lasers, all personnel in the room must wear protective eyewear.

_____ 61. Fire prevention measures must be in place at all times during the use of lasers.

Case Studies

Read the following case studies and answer the questions based on your knowledge of laser surgery and electrosurgery in the surgical technology field.

Case 1: The laser beam can injure tissue other than the site being treated. The laser should not be turned on until the surgeon is ready to start, and it should be turned off as soon as the procedure is completed to avoid the accidental discharge of the laser beam. Areas near the site being treated should be cornered with wet towels to prevent accidental burns. The wet cloth absorbs the laser energy, thus protecting the tissue under the cloth. Flammable paper drapes should not be near the operating field. This material can be set on fire by the laser. All instruments should be anodized to prevent injuries to the patient and surgical personnel. The patient's eyes should be protected at all times.

1. The aforementioned are some protective measures for the patient during the use of laser. List and describe some protective measures for the surgical team.

_____

_____

_____

_____

Case 2: Monopolar electrosurgery—the use of radio frequency (RF) current to cut tissue and control bleeding—has been employed effectively in open operative procedures for over 65 years. In part because of its long history of use in open surgery, it has become the most widely used cutting and coagulation technique in minimally invasive surgery. Though highly versatile, cost effective, and popular, monopolar laparoscopic electrosurgery can compromise patient safety under certain circumstances. The surgeon may directly burn nontargeted internal organs or tissue with the tip of the active electrode through imprecise mechanical operation of a laparoscopic instrument. Stray electrical currents emanating from the laparoscopic instruments can inadvertently burn nontargeted tissues beyond the surgeon's limited field of vision, leading, on occasion, to the patient's death. Such stray energy burns can occur regardless of the surgeon's skill and judgment.

1. List several alternatives to the use of monopolar electrosurgery that may provide less risk for injury to the patient.

_____

_____

_____

_____

Internet Exercise

LASIK is a surgical procedure intended to reduce a person's dependency on glasses or contact lenses. The acronym stands for laser-assisted in situ keratomileusis and is a procedure that permanently changes the shape of the cornea, the clear covering of the front of the eye, using an excimer laser. Using the Internet as a research tool, write a brief paragraph describing this procedure.

_____

_____

_____

_____

_____

Chapter 18
Endoscopic Surgery and Robotics

Key Terms

Write the definition for each term.

1. Adhesions: _____

_____

_____

2. Coupling: _____

_____

_____

3. Endoscope: _____

_____

_____

4. Fiber-optic: _____

_____

_____

5. Hasson cannula: _____

_____

_____

6. Insufflator: _____

_____

_____

7. Monitor: _____

_____

_____

8. Morcelization: _____

_____

_____

9. Objective: _____

_____

_____

10. Ocular: _____

_____

_____

11. Open procedure: _____

_____

_____

12. Pneumoperitoneum: _____

_____

_____

13. Ports: _____

_____

_____

14. Resect: _____

_____

_____

15. Sequential compression devices: _____

_____

_____

16. Trocar and cannula: _____

_____

_____

17. Uterine manipulator: _____

_____

_____

18. Veress needle: _____

_____

_____

Short Answers

19. List the benefits of endoscopic surgery over open procedures.

_____

_____

_____

_____

20. List one difference between open and closed surgery.

_____

_____

_____

_____

21. When the patient has entered the surgical suite, special precautions are taken to minimize risks associated with laparoscopic surgery. List three risks associated with laparoscopic surgery.

_____

_____

_____

_____

22. Explain what is used to prevent embolisms and how they work.

_____

_____

_____

_____

23. The positioning for a patient undergoing an endoscopic procedure depends on the targeted tissues and the patient's physiologic condition. Explain the patient position for pelvic endoscopy.

_____

_____

_____

_____

24. The success of an endoscopic procedure depends on the proper functioning of the equipment. List three problems that may be encountered with equipment during an endoscopic procedure.

_____

_____

_____

_____

25. Every endoscopic procedure has the potential to become an open case. An emergency conversion to open surgery is very rapid. The surgical technologist in the scrub role and the circulator must be prepared for this event. Describe what you would have available if you needed to switch from an endoscopic case to an open case.

_____

_____

_____

_____

26. Identify and describe two techniques used to establish the pneumoperitoneum.

_____

_____

_____

_____

27. When setting up for an endoscopic procedure, the surgical technologist should carefully evaluate all instruments for any damage that may cause them to malfunction during the procedure. List three things that a surgical technologist must look for when examining the endoscope and accessories.

_____

_____

_____

_____

28. Electronic, remote-controlled robotic instruments are under investigation and development. Designed primarily for use during laparoscopic surgery, the robotic arms can hold the endoscope over the target tissue or actually assist in some of the delicate procedures required for the surgery. List the primary benefits of robotic technology.

_____

_____

_____

_____

29. What is the major disadvantage with the use of robotics in distant surgery? What is the cause of this disadvantage?

_____

_____

_____

_____

Matching

Match each term with the correct definition.

A. port

B. veress needle

C. adhesions

D. morcelization

E. pneumoperitoneum

F. trocar and cannula

G. uterine manipulator

H. insufflator

I. Hasson cannula

J. coupling

_____ 30. Cannulated incisions made in the body wall; they receive and stabilize the endoscopic equipment used to perform endoscopic surgery

_____ 31. Instruments inserted through the incision site with a sharp or blunt tip. The tip is inserted through the lumen of the cannula and introduced into the incision site. The trocar is then removed, and the cannula remains in the incision site for the introduction of instruments used for endoscopic procedures

_____ 32. A probelike instrument that is inserted into the distal cervix and used to reposition the uterus during gynecological endoscopic procedures

_____ 33. Scar tissue that binds internal tissues together. This presents a technical problem during endoscopic procedures as it can cause wide variations in the anatomical location of organs

_____ 34. Inflation of the peritoneal cavity with compressed gas such as carbon dioxide so that endoscopic surgery can be performed with decreased risk of trauma to tissues and organs

_____ 35. Electrosurgical contact between two or more instruments during endoscopic surgery; this can result in serious patient burns

_____ 36. A long, slender needle inserted through the abdominal wall to deliver carbon dioxide gas during the creation of the pneumoperitoneum

_____ 37. A process in which tissue is fragmented so it can be withdrawn easily through an endoscopic cannula or suction device

_____ 38. A type of blunt-tipped trocar and cannula assembly used in "open laparoscopy" procedures that is anchored to the body wall with sutures

_____ 39. The device used to deliver carbon dioxide from the tank to the patient to achieve pneumoperitoneum

True/False

Indicate whether the sentence or statement is true (T) or false (F).

_____ 40. Flexible endoscopes are designed for use in tubular structures such as the gastrointestinal tract, genitourinary tract, small ducts, vascular structures, and ear, nasal passages, and sinuses.

_____ 41. The flexible tip of the endoscope cannot be rotated to create a 360° view.

_____ 42. Many flexible endoscope instruments are disposable to prevent the transmission of blood-borne diseases.

_____ 43. The image quality of fiber-optic endoscopes is far superior to that of rigid endoscopes.

_____ 44. The primary use of flexible endoscopy is in diagnostic procedures, although it can be used for tissue dissection and removal.

_____ 45. During endoscopic procedures, it is not important to keep valves and channels flushed.

_____ 46. Following precleaning, the flexible endoscope must be leak tested.

_____ 47. Flexible endoscope accessories such as biopsy forceps or cytology brushes that break the mucous membrane barrier or enter sterile tissue do not need to be sterilized before reuse.

_____ 48. Flexible endoscopes must be stored in a ventilated storage area with the control head secured in an upright position and the distal part of the insertion tube hanging down.

_____ 49. Electrosurgery is used with nearly every type of endoscopic procedure. The risk of patient burns is much higher with endoscopic procedures than with open procedures.

Case Studies

Read the following case studies and answer the questions based on your knowledge of endoscopic surgery and robotics in the surgical technology field.

Case 1: Endoscopy involves the insertion of a scope into various regions of the body for preoperative, intraoperative, and postoperative diagnosis and treatment. The endoscope may be flexible or rigid.

1. Name a surgical procedure that would require a rigid endoscope.

   _____

   _____

   _____

   _____

2. What additional equipment would be needed to perform this procedure?

   _____

   _____

   _____

   _____

3. What risks would be involved with this procedure?

   _____

   _____

   _____

   _____

4. Name a procedure that would use a flexible endoscope.

_____

_____

_____

_____

5. Is this a diagnostic or therapeutic procedure?

_____

_____

_____

_____

Case 2: Tara is a 45-year-old female in good health. She has developed severe pain in her upper-right quadrant about two hours after eating. Tara was admitted to the emergency department and after taking her history and undergoing a physical, she was diagnosed with cholelithiasis and cholecystitis.

1. What is cholelithiasis?

_____

_____

_____

_____

2. What is cholecystitis?

_____

_____

_____

_____

3. What is the cause of cholelithiasis?

_____

_____

_____

_____

4. List three treatment options.

_____

_____

_____

_____

5. Tara's surgeon has scheduled her for a laparoscopic cholecystectomy. Briefly explain the procedure and the specific equipment and instruments that you will need.

_____

_____

_____

_____

Internet Exercise

Robot-assisted surgery is the latest development in endoscopic procedures, a type of minimally invasive surgery, the idea being that less invasive procedures translate into less trauma and postoperative pain for patients. Surgery through smaller incisions typically results in less scarring and faster recovery. Robots are not changing the basics of surgery. Surgeons are still cutting and suturing as they have been for decades. Robots represent a new computer-assisted tool that provides another way for surgeons to work. Using the Internet as a research tool, write a brief paragraph on a specific procedure and a robotic technique used to perform that procedure.

_____

_____

_____

_____

_____

_____

_____

Chapter 19
Diagnostic Procedures

Key Terms

Write the definition for each term.

1. Arterial blood gases (ABGs): _____

_____

_____

2. Biopsy: _____

_____

_____

3. Chemistry studies: _____

_____

_____

4. Complete blood count (CBC): _____

_____

_____

5. Computed tomography (CT): _____

_____

_____

6. Culture and sensitivity (C & S): _____

_____

_____

7. Diagnostic agent: _____

_____

_____

8. Differential count: _____

_____

_____

9. Doppler studies: _____

_____

_____

10. Echocardiography: _____

_____

_____

11. Electrocardiogram (ECG): _____

_____

_____

12. Electrolyte levels: _____

_____

_____

13. Endoscopy: _____

_____

_____

14. Fluoroscopy: _____

_____

_____

15. Frozen section: _____

_____

_____

16. Hematocrit (Hct): _____

_____

_____

17. Hemoglobin (Hb): _____

_____

_____

18. Hemogram: _____

_____

_____

19. History and physical (H & P): _____

_____

_____

20. Magnetic resonance imaging (MRI): _____

_____

_____

21. Positron emission tomography (PET): _____

_____

_____

22. Red blood cell (RBC) count: _____

_____

_____

23. Type and cross (T & C): _____

_____

_____

24. Type and screen (T & S): _____

_____

_____

25. Ultrasound: _____

_____

_____

26. Urinalysis (UA): _____

_____

_____

27. Vital signs: _____

_____

_____

28. White blood cell (WBC) count: _____

_____

_____

29. X-ray: _____

_____

_____

Short Answers

30. What is the purpose of diagnostic procedures and tests?

_____

_____

_____

_____

31. Diagnostic tests and procedures may be considered noninvasive, minimally invasive, or invasive. Define the three categories, and give an example of each.

_____

_____

_____

_____

32. The most common diagnostic procedure involves obtaining the patient's vital signs. Vital signs provide a quick view of the patient's general health. Explain what the four common vital signs access.

_____

_____

_____

_____

33. Why is a patient's history and physical important? List some social or medical problems that could be revealed in a patient's history.

_____

_____

_____

_____

34. Hematology is the study of blood and its cellular components. Essentially, blood is divided into two parts. What are the two parts of blood, and what composes the two parts?

_____

_____

_____

_____

35. Two primary tests are performed to evaluate blood and blood cells in the surgical patient. Identify and describe the two tests.

_____

_____

_____

_____

36. The process of forming a blood clot typically occurs in four stages. Each stage is associated with specific clotting factors that are activated or deactivated as a result of trauma to a blood vessel. Identify and describe the four stages in the process of forming a blood clot.

_____

_____

_____

_____

37. Electrocardiogram is a routine procedure that is performed on anyone over age 40, patients with a personal or family history of cardiac disease, and anyone who has had a previous heart attack or cardiac arrhythmia. Why is electrocardiogram monitoring a standard procedure for all patients in the operating room?

_____

_____

_____

_____

38. Electrocardiography is often used intraoperatively. What is the difference between transthoracic echocardiography and transesophageal echocardiography (TEE)?

_____

_____

_____

_____

39. Describe how time, distance, and shielding can protect the surgical technologist from the adverse effects of radiation.

_____

_____

_____

_____

Matching

Match each term with the correct definition.

A. vital signs

B. type and screen (T & S)

C. arterial blood gases (ABGs)

D. chemistry studies

E. type and cross (T & C)

F. hematocrit (Hct)

G. Doppler studies

H. hemoglobin (Hb)

I. history and physical (H & P)

J. complete blood count (CBC)

_____ 40. A blood test that measures specific components of blood, including hemoglobin, hematocrit, red blood cells, white blood cells and types, platelets, and several blood cell indices

_____ 41. A technique of using ultrasound energy to measure motion within blood vessels

_____ 42. A blood test that uses an arterial blood sample to assess oxygenation and adequacy of ventilation

_____ 43. Various tests that evaluate the presence or levels of certain chemicals within the blood

_____ 44. A test that is used to identify which units of blood match the patient's blood type and their availability if required by the patient

_____ 45. Basic diagnostic indicators that help to immediately assess life-threatening situations

_____ 46. The process of interviewing a patient and conducting a physical examination to assess various anatomical structures and systems

_____ 47. A test that specifically matches a patient's blood with a particular unit or units in the blood bank

_____ 48. A test that examines the percentage of red blood cells as a part of the CBC or hemogram

_____ 49. A test that identifies the capacity of oxygen-carrying cells within the blood

True/False

Indicate whether the sentence or statement is true (T) or false (F).

_____ 50. Diagnostic procedures and techniques are designed to evaluate the entire patient and provide an appropriate plan of care.

_____ 51. A surgical patient with a suspected infection may have samples of tissue or body fluids sent to microbiology to determine the specific type of infectious organism present in the tissue or fluid.

_____ 52. All specimens require some type of fixative.

_____ 53. It is appropriate to pass a specimen off of the sterile field without asking the surgeon's permission.

_____ 54. Neurological monitoring involves the insertion of passive electrodes into the subcutaneous layer of tissue in the extremities and an active electrode that will generate impulses through the spinal cord.

_____ 55. Positron emission tomography imaging is not a good diagnostic tool in determining the location, size, and metabolism of tumors.

_____ 56. An MRI is commonly used to evaluate structures of the brain, muscles, and other connective tissue along the spine.

_____ 57. It is not necessary to wear a lead apron when the fluoroscope is in use during a surgical procedure.

_____ 58. An intraoperative cholangiogram may be requested to rule out the presence of stones within the common bile duct during a cholecystectomy.

_____ 59. Radiopaque solutions are frequently used to assist in the diagnosis of defects or abnormalities of the peripheral vascular, digestive, and urinary systems.

Case Studies

Read the following case studies and answer the questions based on your knowledge of diagnostic procedures in the surgical technology field.

Case 1: Edward, a 7-year-old male, has been brought to the emergency department by his mother. She claims he has been complaining of generalized pain in his lower-right quadrant. She says his appetite has been poor and that he has been running a fever and vomiting.

1. Which structure in the right, lower quadrant might be involved?

   _____

   _____

   _____

   _____

2. List the diagnostic studies that may be performed.

   _____

   _____

   _____

   _____

3. If there is the presence of infection, which diagnostic study will indicate infection?

   _____

   _____

   _____

   _____

4. Which surgical procedure will Edward undergo? Can it be performed laparoscopically?

_____

_____

_____

_____

5. Can Edward sign his own surgical consent? Why or why not?

_____

_____

_____

_____

Case 2: The first case of the day for which you are scrubbing is an abdominal aortic aneurysmectomy.

1. Which diagnostic procedures may the patient have undergone?

_____

_____

_____

_____

2. Which type of anesthesia will be used for this procedure?

_____

_____

_____

_____

3. How will the patient be positioned for this procedure?

_____

_____

_____

_____

4. Would Doppler studies be used during this procedure? If so, for what?

_____

_____

_____

_____

5. If this case had been a ruptured abdominal aneurysm, what would have taken priority during your setup?

_____

_____

_____

_____

Internet Exercise

Intraoperative neuropsychological monitoring has been utilized in an attempt to minimize neurological morbidity from operative manipulations. The goal of such monitoring is to identify changes in brain, spinal cord, and peripheral nerve function prior to irreversible damage. Intraoperative monitoring also has been effective in localizing anatomical structures, including peripheral nerves and the sensor motor cortex, which will help guide the surgeon during the dissection. Using the Internet as a research tool, choose a surgical procedure in which neuromonitoring is used, and write a brief paragraph about how and why it is used during this procedure.

_____

_____

_____

_____

_____

Chapter 20
The Selection of Surgical Instruments

Key Terms

Write the definition for each term.

1. Boggy: _____

   _____

   _____

2. Box lock: _____

   _____

   _____

3. Chisel: _____

   _____

   _____

4. Clamp: _____

   _____

   _____

5. Cross-clamp: _____

   _____

   _____

6. Curettage: _____

   _____

   _____

7. Cutting instrument: _____

_____

_____

8. Dilator: _____

_____

_____

9. Double-action instrument: _____

_____

_____

10. Elevator: _____

_____

_____

11. Friable: _____

_____

_____

12. Fulcrum: _____

_____

_____

13. Hemostat: _____

_____

_____

14. Histology: _____

_____

_____

15. Honed: _____

_____

_____

16. Mixter: _____

_____

_____

17. Points: _____

_____

_____

18. Probe: _____

_____

_____

19. Rongeur: _____

_____

_____

20. Semi-occluding clamp: _____

_____

_____

21. Serosa: _____

_____

_____

22. Shank: _____

_____

_____

23. Tansect: _____

_____

_____

24. Undermine: _____

_____

_____

Short Answers

25. Instrumentation should be learned on a basic level by associating function with design. List three important design features of instrumentation.

_____

_____

_____

_____

26. Why is it important for the surgical technologist not to just "learn the name" of an instrument?

_____

_____

_____

_____

27. Discuss why instruments are assembled in trays.

_____

_____

_____

_____

28. There are three different types of finishes on metal instruments. List the three finishes, and briefly describe each.

_____

_____

_____

_____

29. List the categories of surgical instruments, and give an example of an instrument in each category.

_____

_____

_____

_____

30. List and give examples of different types of tissues. Give an example of a surgical instrument that should be used on the specific type of tissue.

_____

_____

_____

_____

31. Why is the design of the instrument critical in order to perform surgery on different body planes?

_____

_____

_____

_____

32. When anticipating the need for instruments, the surgical technologist should not only consider the body planes but the wound depth as well. Why is the wound depth important?

_____

_____

_____

_____

33. An atraumatic clamp is a type of clamp that is used on delicate tissue that is vascular or easily injured. Describe an atraumatic clamp.

_____

_____

_____

_____

34. Scissors designed to cut tissue should never be used to cut sutures. Explain why this is so.

_____

_____

_____

_____

Matching

Match each term with the correct definition.

A. shank

B. box lock

C. curettage

D. clamp

E. friable

F. elevator

G. hemostat

H. rongeur

I. Mixter

J. cross-clamp

_____ 35. To place one or more clamps at a right angle to an elongated or a tubular structure such as the aorta

_____ 36. The hinge points of surgical instruments

_____ 37. The area of the surgical instrument between the box lock and the finger ring

_____ 38. A nonhinged sharp or dull-tipped instrument, used to separate tissue or to bluntly remodel tissue

_____ 39. Tissue that tears or fragments easily when handled

_____ 40. A hinged instrument with sharp, cup-shaped tips used to extract pieces of bone or other connective tissue

_____ 41. Instrument that is designed to occlude tissue, objects, or fabric between its jaws

_____ 42. To remove tissue by scraping with a surgical curette

_____ 43. A surgical clamp used most commonly to occlude a blood vessel

_____ 44. A type of hemostat with a straight shank and a right-angled tip

True/False

Indicate whether the sentence or statement is true (T) or false (F).

_____ 45. When the surgeon is using a rongeur, it is important to use a damp sponge to keep the tips clean as he or she works.

_____ 46. It is not necessary to keep all tissue cleaned from the instruments as the surgeon works.

_____ 47. The osteotome has two beveled sides; the chisel blade is sloped on one side only.

_____ 48. A brush should be used to keep the blade of the rasp clean as the surgeon is working.

_____ 49. A self-retaining retractor is used to hold the tissue against the walls of the surgical wound by mechanical action.

_____ 50. The needle holder is used to grasp a curved needle during suturing; the length, weight, and type of tip are universal and need not be matched to the suture and tissue.

_____ 51. When removing a scalpel blade from its handle, a heavy needle holder should be used to grasp the blade.

_____ 52. Suctioning instruments are used to suction blood and fluids from the surgical field; they are designed for specific anatomical areas based on function.

_____ 53. A semi-occluding clamp is a traumatic clamp whose jaws come into close contact with each other and place extensive pressure on tissue when applied.

_____ 54. A double-action instrument is one with two hinges in the middle. This provides greater leverage and cutting strength than a single-action instrument.

Case Study

Read the following case study and answer the questions based on your knowledge of the selection of surgical instruments in the surgical technology field.

With the patient in the supine position, a McBurney's incision was made and deepened through the subcutaneous tissue. Using an ESU, the bleeders were cauterized. The external oblique muscle was incised along the length of its fibers using Metzenbaum scissors. The internal oblique and transverse abdominal muscles were bluntly dissected using Kelly clamps. The peritoneum was grasped with two Kelly clamps and raised and nicked with a scalpel. The incision of the peritoneum was completed with Metzenbaum scissors. The appendix was identified, which was grasped with two Babcock clamps and raised into the wound. In addition, another Babcock grasped the cecum, which was mobilized toward the wound. The mesoappendix was serially clamped, divided, and ligated with 2-0 chromic gut suture. The appendiceal base stump was cauterized with an ESU.

The abdominal cavity was irrigated with antibiotic solution. The wound was closed in layers. The peritoneum was closed in a continuous fashion, using 2-0 Maxon suture. The transverse abdominal muscles and internal oblique were closed in an interrupted fashion, using 2-0 Maxon suture. The external oblique aponeurosis was closed in a continuous fashion, using 2-0 Maxon suture, and the skin was closed with staples.

1. Which method of hemostasis was used during incision?

_____

_____

_____

_____

2. Which instrument was used to cut tissue?

_____

_____

_____

_____

3. Why were Babcock clamps used to grasp the appendix and cecum?

_____

_____

_____

_____

4. Which instruments could be used to clamp the appendiceal artery?

_____

_____

_____

_____

5. Will there be a specimen? If so, what will the specimen be?

_____

_____

_____

_____

6. As the surgeon closes the fascia with sutures, which forceps will he or she use?

_____

_____

_____

_____

7. What will the surgical technologist use to keep his or her instruments clean during the case?

_____

_____

_____

_____

8. What is the wound classification?

_____

_____

_____

_____

9. Why is the abdominal cavity irrigated with antibiotic solution?

_____

_____

_____

_____

10. By which other methods could the wound have been closed?

_____

_____

_____

_____

Internet Exercise

As a surgical technologist, you will be responsible for learning the names and uses of many instruments. As the technology in the surgical field continues to change, instruments change as well. Using the Internet as a research tool, choose an instrument and write a brief paragraph describing it, how it is used during surgery, and how it should be cared for.

_____

_____

_____

_____

_____

_____

_____

Chapter 21
General Surgery

SECTION I: **INCISIONS**
SECTION II: **HERNIAS**
SECTION III: **GASTROINTESTINAL SURGERY**
SECTION IV: **SURGERY OF THE BILIARY SYSTEM, LIVER, PANCREAS, AND SPLEEN**
SECTION V: **BREAST SURGERY**

Key Terms

Write the definition for each term.

1. Abdominal peritoneum: _____

   _____

   _____

2. Epigastric: _____

   _____

   _____

3. Fascia: _____

   _____

   _____

4. Subcutaneous tissue: _____

   _____

   _____

5. Paramedian: _____

   _____

   _____

6. Linea alba: _____

_____

_____

7. Muscle-splitting incision: _____

_____

_____

8. Hypogastric: _____

_____

_____

9. Indirect inguinal hernia: _____

_____

_____

10. Direct inguinal hernia: _____

_____

_____

11. Total extraperitoneal (TEP) surgical approach: _____

_____

_____

12. Ventral hernia: _____

_____

_____

13. Anastomosis: _____

_____

_____

14. Bilroth II procedure: _____

_____

15. Exploratory laparotomy: _____

_____

_____

16. GERD: _____

_____

_____

17. NG tube: _____

_____

_____

18. PEG tube: _____

_____

_____

19. Parenchyma: _____

_____

_____

20. Pancreatojejunostomy: _____

_____

_____

21. Glisson's capsule: _____

_____

_____

22. Trisegmentectomy: _____

_____

_____

23. Frozen section: _____

_____

_____

24. Lumpectomy: _____

_____

_____

25. Palpable: _____

_____

_____

26. Undermine: _____

_____

_____

27. Tylectomy: _____

_____

_____

Labeling

28. Label the following:

29. Label the following:

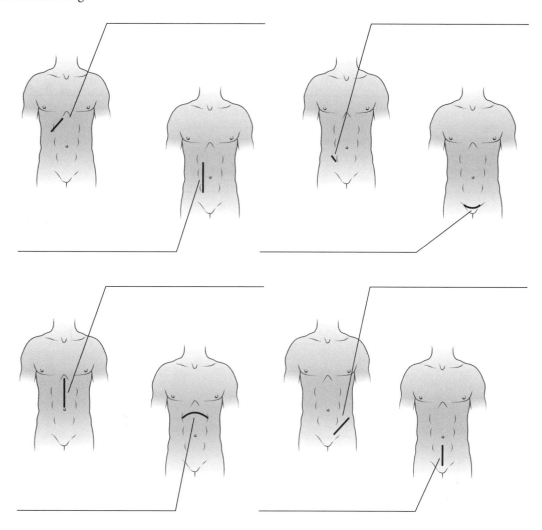

Short Answers

30. Discuss the difference in the anatomy between direct and indirect hernias.

_____

_____

_____

_____

31. Why is it important to do a full instrument count for an inguinal hernia repair?

_____

_____

_____

_____

32. Describe a therapeutic procedure.

_____

_____

_____

_____

33. Describe the method for clean closure during a "GI" or dirty case.

_____

_____

_____

_____

34. Your patient is scheduled for an appendectomy. You are setting up your Mayo stand. Please draw your instruments (and label them) on the Mayo stand. Do not choose more than 12 instruments or pieces of equipment to put on your Mayo stand.

35. Draw and label the large bowel, including all five distinct areas, the flexures, and the appendix.

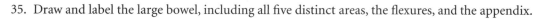

Labeling

36. Label the following:

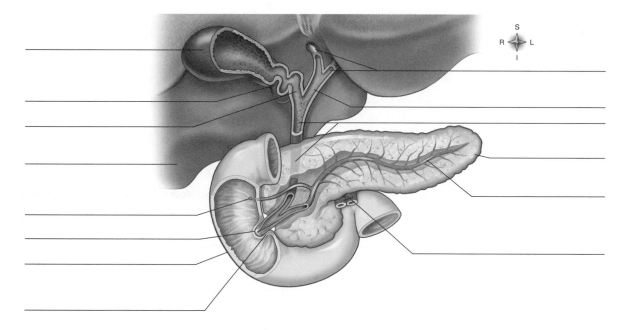

37. Label the following:

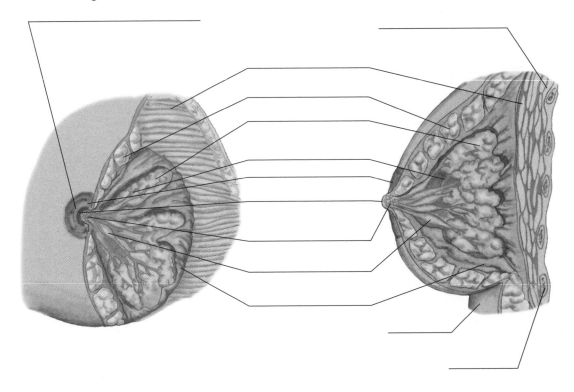

Short Answers

38. Which type of dressing is needed following a breast biopsy? Why?

_____

_____

_____

_____

39. Discuss the psychological considerations that might be needed by a mastectomy patient as she is entering the operating room.

_____

_____

_____

_____

40. Your patient is an A.M. admit. She is scheduled for a left simple mastectomy. She has staples at the left infra-areolar area where a breast biopsy was done three days ago.

    A. The biopsy results were positive for ductal cancer in situ. What does this mean?

    _____

    _____

    _____

    _____

    B. What special considerations will you (as the scrub tech) need to address in preparation for her operation?

    _____

    _____

    _____

    _____

41. Your surgical patient is scheduled for a left breast biopsy and a right simple mastectomy. Which procedure will you do first? Why?

    _____

    _____

    _____

    _____

Internet Exercises

1. Do an Internet search to find a professional organization that is associated with the profession of surgical technology. Once you find the home page, look for a journal article from *Surgical Technology Magazine,* and find an article from the archives dealing with any general surgical procedure. Once you have read the article, write a short, one-page review.

   Rate the article using a scale of 1–10 (1 = poor and 10 = excellent). In your report, include a short critique and a rating for each of the following areas:

   A. How easy was it for you to read through the medical terminology?

   B. Did the author include information specific to a surgical technologist (such as setup, instrumentation, or anatomy)?

   C. Did the author include a step-by-step description that would enhance your knowledge about the procedure?

   D. What did you learn by doing this research that you did not previously know?

2. Conduct an Internet search on the difference between a traditional Roux-en-Y (which was typically done for cancer) and the new bariatrics procedure for weight loss.

   A. Write a paragraph on each of the procedures.

   B. Discuss the differences involved in the anatomy.

   C. Discuss the differences involved in the suturing/stapling techniques.

Chapter 22
Gynecological and Obstetrical Surgery

Key Terms

Write the definition for each term.

1. Ablate: _____

_____

2. Adnexa: _____

_____

3. Cerclage: _____

_____

4. Cystocele: _____

_____

5. Dermoid cyst: _____

_____

6. Electrolytic media: _____

_____

7. En bloc: _____

_____

8. Endometriosis: _____

_____

9. Fibroid: _____

_____

10. Fulguration: _____

_____

11. Glycine: _____

_____

12. Hyperplasia: _____

_____

13. Hysteroscopy: _____

_____

14. Incompetent cervix: _____

_____

15. Incomplete abortion: _____

_____

16. LEEP: _____

_____

17. Leiomyoma: _____

_____

18. Missed abortion: _____

_____

19. Nonelectrolytic media: _____

_____

20. Obturator: _____

_____

21. Patency: _____

_____

22. Perineum: _____

_____

23. Photothermal ablation: _____

_____

24. PID: _____

_____

25. Rectocele: _____

_____

26. Reflection: _____

_____

27. Retrograde: _____

_____

28. Shirodkar's procedure: _____

_____

29. Sorbitol: _____

_____

30. Transcervically: _____

_____

Labeling

31. Label the illustration using the following terms:

fundus of the uterus	ovarian ligament	endometrium
body of the uterus	broad ligament	myometrium
ovary	uterine artery and vein	external os of vaginal cervical
fimbriae	vagina	

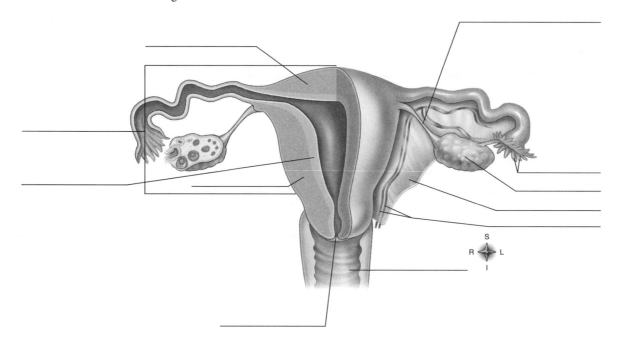

32. Label the following anatomical picture of the internal female genitalia:

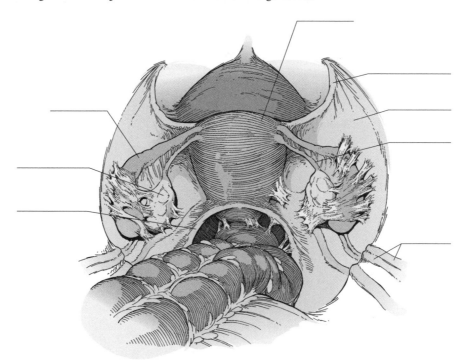

33. Label the following anatomical picture of the external female genitalia:

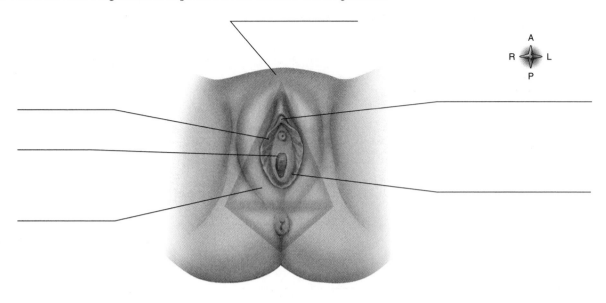

Short Answers

34. Describe the difference between rectocele and cystocele. _____

    A. Rectocele:

    _____

    _____

    B. Cystocele:

    _____

    _____

35. List all of the ligaments of the uterus and ovaries.

    _____

    _____

    _____

36. Draw a picture of the pregnant uterus with a fetus in normal presentation and the placenta previa.

37. Describe the difference between placenta previa and placenta abruptio.

_____

_____

_____

38. Describe the advantages to laparoscopic versus open procedures in OB/GYN procedures.

_____

_____

_____

39. Define the following types of medical abortions:

    A. A *missed abortion:*

    _____

    _____

    B. An *incomplete abortion:*

    _____

    _____

C. An *imminent abortion:*

_____

_____

40. What is CPD?

_____

_____

_____

41. Name four fetal presentations that might result in a C-section delivery.

_____

_____

_____

42. Define *menometrorrhagia.*

_____

_____

_____

43. Define *menorrhagia.*

_____

_____

_____

44. What is a uterine leiomyoma?

_____

_____

_____

45. Describe the difference between a Wertheim procedure and TAH.

_____

_____

_____

46. Describe three different types of sterilization methods that might be employed through the laparoscope.

_____

_____

_____

47. What is another name for a dermoid cyst?

_____

_____

_____

Internet Exercises

1. Go to any search engine on the Internet and search for operating room nursing and surgical technology. Once a site is found, search the site for journal articles and check the archives for procedures dealing with OB/GYN and answer the following questions:

    A. Name of the site found: _____

    B. How is the site associated with their future profession? _____

    _____

    C. List the names of the procedures found (minimum of 10) as well as the web page on which the article was found.

    _____

    _____

    _____

    _____

    _____

    D. Choose one of the 10 procedures found and read the article.

    E. Critique the article for the following: content, readability, significance to the surgical technologist, instrumentation described in the article, medications specific to OB/GYN procedures listed in the article.

2. Research online total abdominal hysterectomy and HRT (hormone replacement therapy) and answer the following questions:

   A. Is the information easily found for patients who might be looking to educate themselves about HRT?

   _____

   B. Which drugs are involved in HRT?

   _____

   _____

   C. What are the benefits of HRT?

   _____

   _____

   D. What problems are associated with HRT?

   _____

   _____

   E. List the website used as well as the journal article.

   _____

   _____

3. Look up stem cell research on the Internet. Once you have found several sites to reference, answer the following questions about stem cells:

   A. Are fetal cells the only source for stem cells?

   _____

   B. What are stem cells currently used for?

   _____

   _____

   C. Is there a difference between stem cell use in the United States and in other countries?

   _____

   _____

D. What is your opinion about stem cell research and stem cell usage now that you have researched the sources and uses of the cells?

_____

_____

_____

_____

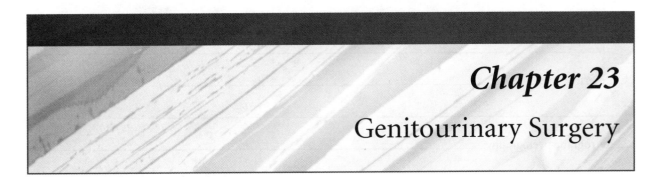

Chapter 23
Genitourinary Surgery

Key Terms

Write the definition for each term.

1. BPH: _____

_____

2. Calculi: _____

_____

3. Circumcision: _____

_____

4. Epispadias: _____

_____

5. ESWL: _____

_____

6. Hematuria: _____

_____

7. Hypospadias: _____

_____

8. Hypothermia: _____

_____

9. Lithotripsy: _____

_____

10. Nonelectrolytic: _____

_____

11. Resectoscope: _____

_____

12. Retrograde pyelography: _____

_____

13. Stent: _____

_____

14. Tamponade: _____

_____

15. Torsion: _____

_____

16. Transurethral: _____

_____

17. TURBT: _____

18. TURP: _____

19. UTI: _____

Labeling

20. Label the illustration using the following terms:

renal artery   ureter   cortex
renal vein   renal pelvis   medulla
hilus   calyx

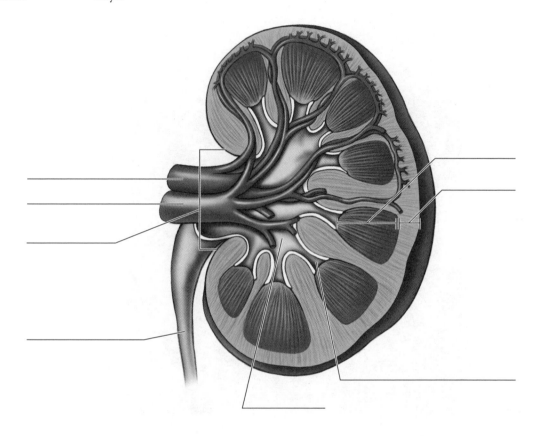

21. Label the illustration using the following terms:

urinary bladder	prepuce	anus
vas deferens	seminal vesicle	epididymis
urethra	ejaculatory duct	testis
penis	prostate gland	scrotum
glans penis	bulbourethral gland	

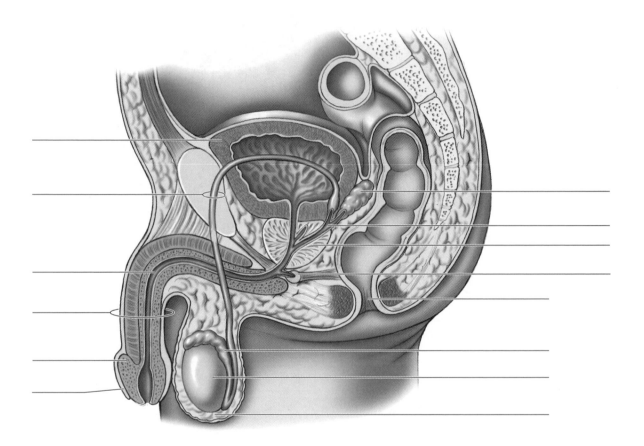

Short Answers

22. There are generally three basic approaches to the genitourinary system. Name them, and briefly describe each approach.

_____

_____

_____

23. Urinary procedures are classified as *open* or *closed*. Describe what is involved in both types of procedures.

_____

_____

_____

24. Each kidney is covered by three separate tissue layers that protect it from injury and also help hold it in place. Name each tissue layer and its function.

_____

_____

_____

25. In a previous exercise you labeled a drawing of the human kidney. Now go back to that drawing and sketch the adrenal glands into their proper place.

_____

_____

_____

26. What is the major difference between the male and the female urethra?

_____

_____

_____

27. What are the six main lobes of the prostate?

_____

_____

_____

28. Extreme hazards are associated with the use of electrosurgical procedures in the presence of fluids. Which procedures (in this unit) require the use of the ESU and continuous irrigation?

_____

_____

_____

29. Name the six uses of urinary drainage systems, as listed in the text.

_____

_____

_____

30. Name a GU procedure that would require the short-term use of a urinary catheter.

_____

_____

_____

31. Name a GU procedure that would require a urinary catheter for the maintenance of continuity of the urethra.

_____

_____

_____

32. Explain why a surgeon would place a *stent* as opposed to a urinary drainage catheter.

_____

_____

_____

33. During most closed GU procedures, the bladder is distended with solution. Which solutions should be used?

_____

_____

_____

34. What temperature should the irrigation be during a cystoscopy? Why?

_____

_____

_____

35. Name three guidelines for the care and handling of a cystoscope.

_____

_____

_____

36. What is the goal of cystourethroscopy (cystoscopy)?

_____

_____

_____

37. What causes the formation of bladder stones?

_____

_____

_____

38. What is a varicocele, and what causes its formation?

_____

_____

_____

39. Why would an adult need a circumcision?

_____

_____

_____

40. How does a surgical technologist care for the specimen from a pyelolithotomy?

_____

_____

_____

41. Your patient is going to the OR for a diagnostic cystoscopy. He has had symptoms that have facilitated this procedure. List his potential symptoms.

_____

_____

_____

42. List the basic instrument setup needed for a cystoscopy.

A. _____   L. _____

B. _____   M. _____

C. _____   N. _____

D. _____   O. _____

E. _____   P. _____

F. _____   Q. _____

G. _____   R. _____

H. _____   S. _____

I. _____   T. _____

J. _____   U. _____

K. _____

Internet Exercises

1. Use the Internet to prepare for a discussion about prostate surgery. Search for a site discussing prostate cancer such as the Urological Research Foundation or the National Bladder Foundation. Find answers to the following possible patient questions:

   A. If I have a TURP will I be incontinent of urine following the operation?

   _____

   _____

   B. One year ago my PSA was 1.83, now it is 2.78. Is this rising too fast for a 53-year-old?

   _____

   _____

   C. If I have cancer of the prostate, how serious is this cancer?

   _____

   _____

   D. How long will it take to recover from this surgery?

   _____

   _____

   E. Can I still be sexually active following a TURP?

   _____

   _____

   F. How common are prostate calculi?

   _____

   _____

Chapter 24
Ophthalmic Surgery

Key Terms

Write the definition for each term.

1. Aqueous humor: _____

_____

2. Bridle suture: _____

_____

3. Buckling component: _____

_____

4. Capsulorrhexis: _____

_____

5. Cataract: _____

_____

6. Choroid: _____

_____

7. Conformer: _____

_____

8. Conjunctiva: _____

_____

9. Cryotherapy: _____

_____

10. Diathermy: _____

_____

11. Enucleation: _____

_____

12. Evisceration: _____

_____

13. Exenteration: _____

_____

14. Glaucoma: _____

_____

15. Globe: _____

_____

16. Hydroxyapatite implant: _____

_____

17. Keratoplasty: _____

_____

18. Phacoemulsification: _____

_____

19. Posterior chamber: _____

_____

20. Pterygium: _____

_____

21. Trabeculectomy: _____

_____

22. Vitreous humor: _____

_____

Labeling

23. Label the illustration using the following terms:

lacrimal canals	puncta	lacrimal ducts
lacrimal sac	nasolacrimal duct	lacrimal gland
caruncle		

24. Label the illustration using the following terms:

optic nerve	choroid	anterior chamber	lens
central artery and vein	retina	iris	pupil
posterior chamber	ciliary body	cornea	lacrimal caruncle
sclera	lower lid	visual axis	optic disc

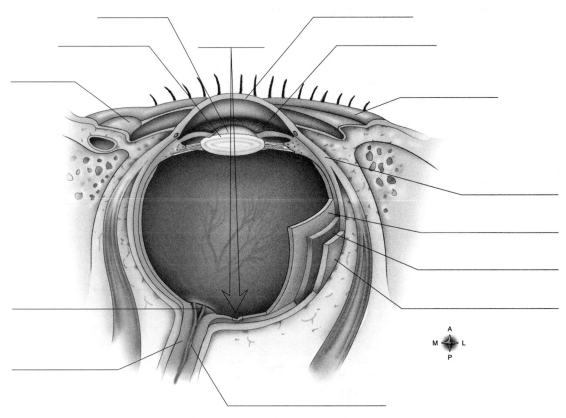

Short Answers

25. Name and discuss the 5 types of anesthetic used for an ophthalmic patient.

A. _____

_____

B. _____

_____

C. _____

_____

D. _____

_____

E. _____

_____

26. Why is verification of the operative site such a big part of preoperative care for a surgical ophthalmic patient? Discuss who has the ultimate responsibility of verification of the operative site.

_____

_____

_____

_____

_____

27. Your surgical patient is a 4-year-old girl. She is in the operating room and under general anesthesia. Your surgeon has started the procedure and has asked you for a "bridal suture." You do not have one, so you ask your circulator to get one for you.

A. Which type of suture do you ask for?

_____

_____

B. Why does your surgeon want the suture?

_____

_____

C. List 10 guidelines to follow when handling the microscope.

1. _____

2. _____

3. _____

4. _____

5. _____

6. _____

7. _____

8. _____

9. _____

10. _____

Medications

Research the medication classifications and fill in the table below:

Classification of medication	Action on the patient	Name of one medication in this class
28. Local anesthetic		
29. Antibiotic		
30. Anti-inflammatory		
31. Diagnostic agent		
32. Enzymatic		
33. Irrigant		
34. Mitotic		
35. Mydriatic		

Internet Exercises

1. Research the LASIK procedure on the Internet for the following information:

   A. If you were a patient, in the state in which you are attending school, where could you go for the surgery?

   _____

   B. How far would you have to travel to get the operation done?

   _____

   C. How much would the surgery cost?

   _____

   D. Will your insurance pay for the surgery?

   _____

   E. Is there an age limit for the surgery?

   _____

F. Who is qualified to perform the operation in your state?

_____

G. Who is qualified to perform the operation in other countries?

_____

2. Go to Cornea-Genetic Eye Medical Institute at Cedars-Sinai Medical Center and research corneal transplants.

   A. Which conditions may require corneal transplants?

   _____

   _____

   B. What can the patient expect after transplant surgery?

   _____

   _____

   C. What complications can occur?

   _____

   _____

   D. Who is best qualified to perform a corneal transplant?

   _____

   E. Find the section on Pediatric Corneal Transplantation, and read the information from the website to answer the following questions:

   F. Why would a child or infant need a corneal transplant?

   _____

   _____

   G. How many pediatric corneal procedures are performed annually?

   _____

Chapter 25
Otorhinolaryngologic, Oral, and Maxillofacial Surgery

Key Terms

Write the definition for each term.

1. Canalplasty: _____

   _____

2. Cholesteatoma: _____

   _____

3. Effusion: _____

   _____

4. Hyperkeratotic: _____

   _____

5. Keratin: _____

   _____

6. Maxillomandibular fixation: _____

   _____

7. Mucocele: _____

   _____

8. Nasal polyp: _____

   _____

9. Neoplasm: _____

_____

10. Osteotomy: _____

_____

11. Otitis media: _____

_____

12. Otorrhea: _____

_____

13. Ototoxic: _____

_____

14. Perichondrium: _____

_____

15. Pharyngitis: _____

_____

16. Tracheotomy: _____

_____

17. Turbinectomy: _____

_____

18. Tympanoplasty: _____

_____

19. Uvulopalatopharyngoplasty: _____

_____

SURGERY OF THE EAR

Labeling

20. Label the following:

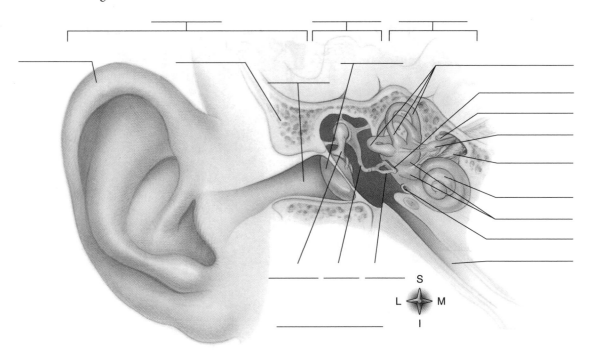

21. Label the following:

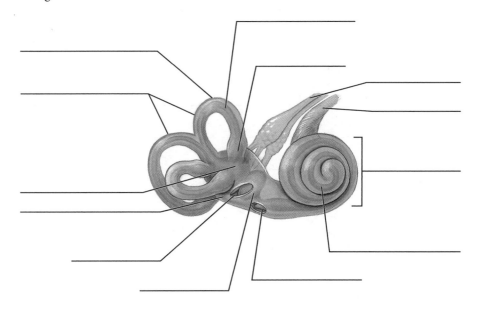

Short Answers

22. Identify the instrument set pictured below. _____

_____

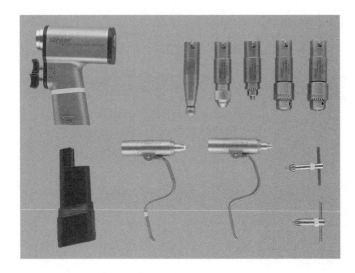

23. Describe the standard operating lenses used in ENT surgery.

_____

_____

_____

_____

24. Describe the prep and drape used in ENT surgery.

_____

_____

_____

_____

25. Describe the two types of hearing loss and what causes each type of loss.

_____

_____

_____

_____

SURGERY OF THE NOSE, THROAT, AND MOUTH

Labeling

26. Label the following:

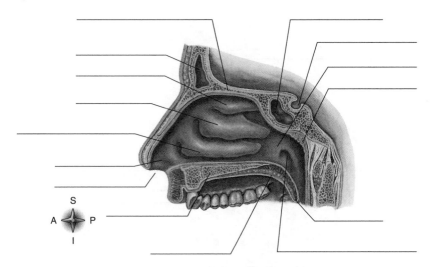

27. Label the following picture of the anatomy of the larynx:

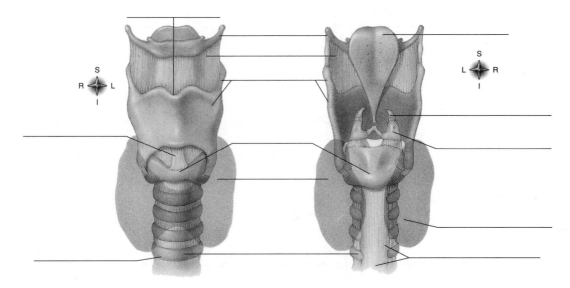

Short Answers

28. Describe the pharynx and its three distinct areas of anatomy.

_____

_____

_____

_____

29. When are sinus scopes used? Describe them.

_____

_____

_____

_____

Medications

Describe the following types of medications and how they are utilized in ENT surgical procedures.

30. Local: _____

_____

31. Epinephrine: _____

_____

32. Cocaine: _____

_____

33. Decongestant: _____

_____

34. Bismuth: _____

_____

SURGERY OF THE HEAD AND NECK

Short Answers

35. Describe why a patient would be put on a doughnut or a Mayfield headrest for ENT procedures.

_____

_____

_____

_____

36. Name the three reasons for performing a laryngectomy.

A. _____

B. _____

_____

C. _____

MAXILLOFACIAL TRAUMA AND ORAL SURGERY

Labeling

37. Label the following:

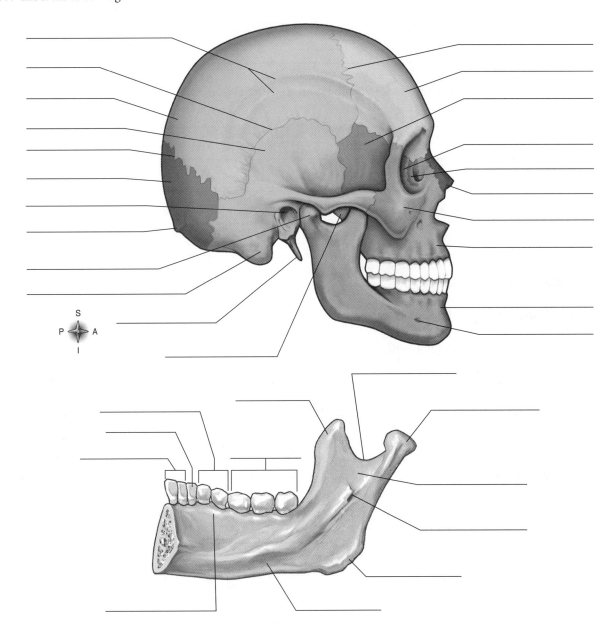

Internet Exercises

1. Research thyroidectomy on the Internet and then answer the following questions from your research. What can your patient find out about thyroidectomy from the Internet?

   A. Can your patient find step-by-step procedure information on the Internet site you chose? Did you?

   _____

   _____

   _____

   B. Does the Internet site list potential postoperative complications for patients to find? List them.

   _____

   _____

   _____

   C. List five of your Internet reference sites and what you learned from each.

   _____

   _____

   _____

   _____

   _____

2. Research cochlear implants on the Internet.

   A. Go to the Cochlear Implant Association and answer the following questions:

      1. What is a cochlear implant?

      _____

      _____

      _____

      2. How does one educate a child who has a cochlear implant?

      _____

      _____

      _____

3. How does one choose a cochlear implant center?

_____

_____

_____

Chapter 26
Plastic and Reconstructive Surgery

Key Terms

Write the definition for each term.

1. Aesthetic: _____

_____

2. Augmentation: _____

_____

3. Autograft: _____

_____

4. Conjunctival sulcus: _____

_____

5. Deepithelialized: _____

_____

6. Eschar: _____

_____

7. Hydrodressing: _____

_____

8. Imbricate: _____

_____

9. Philtrum: _____

_____

10. Photo damage: _____

_____

11. Plicate: _____

_____

12. Pretrichial: _____

_____

13. Ptosis: _____

_____

14. Supratarsal crease: _____

_____

15. Turgid: _____

_____

Labeling

16. Label the following:

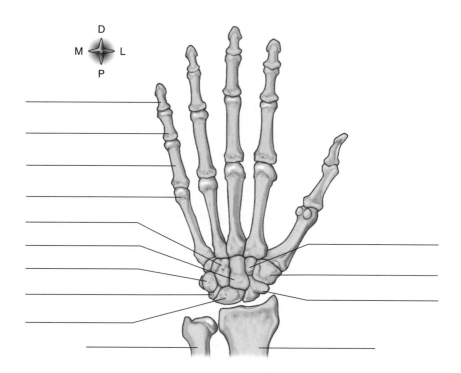

17. Label the following:

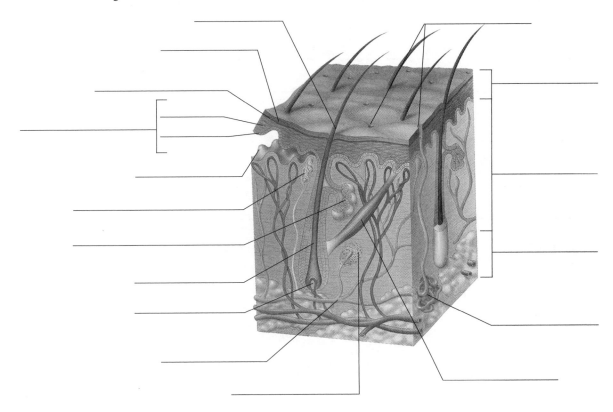

Short Answers

18. Discuss the difference between deepithelialization and debridement.

_____

_____

_____

19. Differentiate between STSG and FTSG by placing an S (for STSG) or an F (for FTSG) next to each of the following statements.

_____ 1. Consist of the epidermis and a portion of the papillary dermis

_____ 2. Consist of the entire epidermis and dermis

_____ 3. The surgeon will use a dermatome for this type of graft

_____ 4. The donor site will have to be sutured closed with this type of graft

_____ 5. The donor site will leave a linear scar from the incision

_____ 6. The donor site will be covered with

20. List the significant complications for your patient who is undergoing a liposuction.

_____

_____

_____

21. Describe the patient who is an excellent candidate for liposuction.

_____

_____

_____

22. Research the types of sutures that are typically used by the plastic surgeons in your area and then answer the following:

    A. What is the typical closure for skin on the patient's face?

        1. Needle type:

_____

_____

        2. Size of the suture:

_____

_____

        3. Type of suture material:

_____

_____

23. How are the sutures used on the patient's face the same or different from the sutures that the plastic surgeon might use on a syndactyly repair?

_____

_____

_____

24. Describe the specific anatomy that is found in the epidermis.

_____

_____

_____

25. Describe the specific anatomy that is found in the dermis.

_____

_____

_____

26. Name the eight carpal bones. _____

    A. _____

    B. _____

    C. _____

    D. _____

    E. _____

    F. _____

    G. _____

    H. _____

27. Make up a mnemonic device to help you remember the eight carpal bones:

    A. T _____

    B. T _____

    C. C _____

    D. H _____

    E. S _____

    F. L _____

    G. T _____

    H. P _____

28. The principles of laser safety must be adhered to during laser procedures. Laser safety was discussed in Chapter 17. To refresh your memory, list four laser safety practices.

A. _____

B. _____

C. _____

D. _____

29. List four laser safety practices that would be used to protect your patient.

A. _____

B. _____

C. _____

D. _____

30. Describe the different types of implants that might be used in facial operations.

_____

_____

_____

31. Explain the term *demarcation.*

_____

_____

_____

32. Research the prep solution alcohol, and report any contraindications for its use in plastic surgery facial procedures.

_____

_____

_____

33. Research the prep solution Betadine, and report any contraindications for its use in plastic surgery facial procedures.

_____

_____

_____

34. Research the prep solution Hibiclens, and report any contraindications for its use in plastic surgery facial procedures.

_____

_____

_____

35. Research the prep solution Phisohex, and report any contraindications for its use in plastic surgery facial procedures.

_____

_____

_____

36. Research the terms *allograft* and *homograft* and their possible uses in plastic surgical procedures.

_____

_____

_____

37. What are the major functional differences between the two lower lid blepharoplasties?

_____

_____

_____

38. Draw a picture of a near pedicle graft from a forehead to repair a nasal defect. Include in your drawing labels for the following: donor site, recipient site, and suture used.

39. Describe a rotation flap.

_____

_____

_____

40. Describe a composite flap.

_____

_____

_____

41. Describe a first-degree burn.

_____

_____

_____

42. Describe a second-degree burn.

_____

_____

_____

43. Describe a third-degree burn.

_____

_____

_____

44. Describe syndactyly.

_____

_____

_____

45. What types of grafting measures are used in syndactyly repair?

_____

_____

_____

46. What are the two reasons a patient may choose to have a mammoplasty?

_____

_____

_____

47. Explain how a cleft lip occurs.

_____

_____

_____

48. Explain how a cleft palate occurs.

_____

_____

_____

49. If your pediatric patient has microtia, how would reconstruction be performed and at what age?

_____

_____

_____

Internet Exercises

1. Go to any plastic surgery site and research the pros and cons of Botox injections.

    A. What can the patient expect as far as the treatment is concerned?

    _____

    _____

    1. Where is the procedure done? _____

    2. Is the procedure painful? _____

    3. What is the postoperative recovery phase? _____

    _____

4. How long do the results take before the Botox takes effect? _____

5. Is there any bruising? _____

6. When will the patient have to repeat the injections? _____

7. What is the cost of the injections? _____

B. Research the medication used.

1. What is the medication used in Botox injections? _____

_____

2. What is the history of the drug? _____

_____

3. What is the drug classification? _____

4. How much of the medication is used in the injections? _____

5. Are there any complications from the treatments? _____

_____

6. In your opinion, are these treatments safe? _____

_____

7. List your Internet research sites. _____

_____

2. Your surgical patient, Mrs. Smith, is scheduled for a mastectomy for DCIS. Research this type of cancer on the Internet and report your findings by answering the following questions:

A. What type of cancer does Mrs. Smith have?

_____

B. If Mrs. Smith chooses to have a mastectomy, which type of reconstructive procedures can be done the same day of her mastectomy?

_____

C. Research and state your patient's prognosis if she has a nipple graft and is a cigarette smoker. (This question relates to the reconstruction only and not the prognosis of the cancer.)

_____

D. Why is cigarette smoking a contraindication for skin grafting?

_____

E. List your Internet research sites.

_____

_____

Chapter 27
Orthopedic Surgery

Key Terms

Write the definition for each term.

1. Acetabulum: _____

_____

2. Allograft: _____

_____

3. Amputation: _____

_____

4. Ankylosis: _____

_____

5. Arthritis: _____

_____

6. Arthrocentesis: _____

_____

7. Arthrodesis: _____

_____

8. Arthrogram: _____

_____

9. Arthroplasty: _____

_____

10. Arthroscopy: _____

_____

11. Arthrotomy: _____

_____

12. Articulation: _____

_____

13. Baker's cyst: _____

_____

14. Bursa: _____

_____

15. Cardiac muscle: _____

_____

16. C-arm: _____

_____

17. Contracture: _____

_____

18. Electromyogram: _____

_____

19. Epiphysiodesis: _____

_____

20. Exostosis: _____

_____

21. Exsanguination: _____

_____

22. Fascia: _____

_____

23. Fasciotomy: _____

_____

24. Fracture: _____

_____

25. Gout: _____

_____

26. Hematopoiesis: _____

_____

27. Joint cavity: _____

_____

28. Joint mouse: _____

_____

29. Ligament: _____

_____

30. Neuropathy: _____

_____

31. Osteoarthritis: _____

_____

32. Osteoarthrotomy: _____

_____

33. Osteoblast: _____

_____

34. Osteogenesis: _____

_____

35. Osteomalacia: _____

_____

36. Osteomyelitis: _____

_____

37. Osteonecrosis: _____

_____

38. Osteosclerosis: _____

_____

39. Osteotomy: _____

_____

40. Patella: _____

_____

41. Sesamoid: _____

_____

42. Smooth muscle: _____

_____

43. Striated muscle: _____

_____

44. Suture: _____

_____

45. Symphysis: _____

_____

46. Synchondrosis: _____

_____

47. Syndesmosis: _____

_____

48. Tendon: _____

_____

49. Traction: _____

_____

Labeling

50. Label the illustration using the following terms:

diaphysis   yellow marrow   spongy bone   compact bone
articulating cartilage   periosteum   epiphyseal plate   medullary cavity
endosteum   epiphysis   red marrow cavities

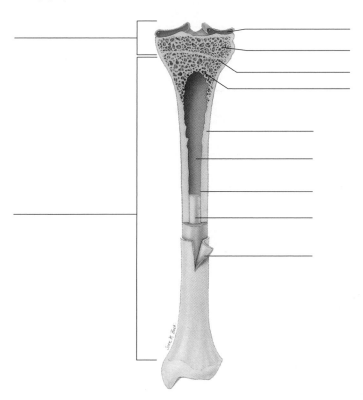

Matching

Match the medical terminology that describes movement with its correct definition.

A. eversion   _____ 51. To take away from; away from midline

B. adduction   _____ 52. To move toward the midline

C. abduction   _____ 53. To turn outward

D. flexion   _____ 54. Forward movement

E. volar   _____ 55. Backward movement

F. varus   _____ 56. Bent outward or twisted, away from the midline of the body

G. extension   _____ 57. Turned inward

H. valgus   _____ 58. Palm of the hand or the sole of the foot; also called palmar or palmaris
                              or volaris

Definitions

Define the following anatomical terminology that describes bone.

59. Crest: _____

60. Spine: _____

61. Condyle: _____

62. Process: _____

63. Tubercle: _____

64. Tuberosity: _____

65. Foramen: _____

66. Sinus: _____

67. Sulcus: _____

Short Answers

Describe the difference between the following:

68. Nonunion fracture: _____

_____

69. Malunion fracture: _____

_____

70. Delayed union fracture: _____

_____

71. Name the 3 phases of fracture healing: _____

_____

_____

72. Name 5 possible complications of fractures and fracture management: _____

A. _____

B. _____

C. _____

D. _____

E. _____

Internet Exercises

1. Go to your favorite search engine and type in orthopedic implants. Once you settle on a site, see if it has a patient information section. Conduct a thorough search of the site, and answer the following questions:

A. Did the site chosen provide patient information about different conditions?

_____

B. Did the site chosen provide patient information on alternate treatments, or did it jump right into surgery?

_____

C. Did the site chosen "speak" to the patient in terms he or she could understand, or was it very technical?

_____

Return to the home page, and answer the following questions (you may need to expand your search):

D. Did the site chosen have a special "surgeon's" corner? If so, which type of information was available to the surgeon?

_____

_____

E. Did the site chosen contain case studies of actual patients and their results?

_____

F. Did the site chosen describe the failure rate of different prosthesis?

_____

G. List the Internet sites used.

_____

_____

2. Go to your favorite search engine and research the rehabilitation that a patient would go through who has just undergone an open ACL repair. You may need to look at sites specific to physical therapy rather than orthopedic procedures. Once you find the site, do a search, and answer the following questions:

   A. How long is the rehabilitation period for a patient who has undergone an ACL?

   _____

   B. Which type of rehabilitation is needed for the patient?

   _____

   C. What will happen if the patient does *not* undergo the rehabilitation as prescribed?

   _____

   D. Who designs the rehabilitation for the patient, the surgeon or the physical therapist?

   _____

   E. Does insurance pay for the rehabilitation?

   _____

Chapter 28
Peripheral Vascular Surgery

Key Terms

Write the definition for each term.

1. Angioplasty: _____

_____

2. Arteriosclerosis: _____

_____

3. Arteriotomy: _____

_____

4. Arteriovenous fistula: _____

_____

5. Atherosclerosis: _____

_____

6. Bifurcation: _____

_____

7. Diastolic pressure: _____

_____

8. Doppler duplex ultrasonography: _____

_____

9. Electroencephalogram (EEG): _____

_____

10. Embolus: _____

_____

11. Endarterectomy: _____

_____

12. Etiology: _____

_____

13. Extracorporeal: _____

_____

14. Hemodialysis: _____

_____

15. Infarction: _____

_____

16. In situ: _____

_____

17. Intravascular ultrasound: _____

_____

18. Ischemia: _____

_____

19. Lumen: _____

_____

20. Percutaneous: _____

_____

21. Stent: _____

_____

22. Systolic pressure: _____

_____

23. Thrombus: _____

_____

24. Tunica adventitia: _____

_____

Labeling

25. Label the illustration using the following terms:

right pulmonary veins	left pulmonary veins	inferior vena cava
right pulmonary artery	left atrium	right atrium
pulmonary trunk	left ventricle	superior vena cava
left pulmonary artery	aorta	pulmonary circulation

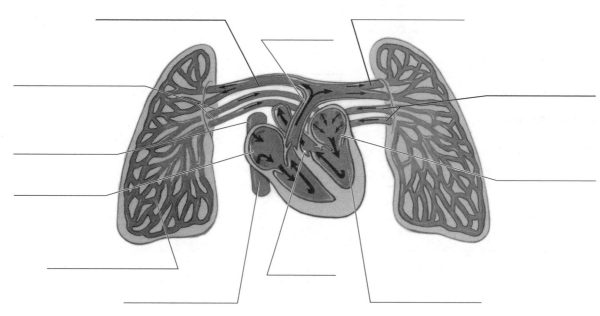

26. Label the illustration using the following list of terms:

tunica intima   venous valve   tunica externa
basement membrane   tunica media   endothelium

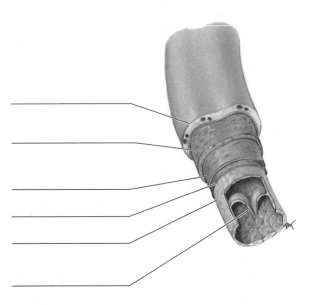

Short Answers

27. Describe the difference between veins and arteries.

_____

_____

_____

_____

28. Describe the tissue layers of blood vessels.

_____

_____

_____

_____

29. Describe the difference between the systemic vascular system and the pulmonary vascular system.

   _____

   _____

   _____

30. Name four characteristics of vascular suture as described in the text.

   A. _____

   B. _____

   C. _____

   D. _____

31. Vascular grafts are used to replace a blood vessel or to make a patch. Describe the three types of grafts listed in the text.

   A. _____

   B. _____

   C. _____

32. Explain atherosclerosis.

   _____

   _____

   _____

33. When removing plaque from an artery, there is a risk of breaking it apart and causing an embolus. Describe what effects an embolus might have on your surgical patient who is undergoing a carotid endarterectomy.

   _____

   _____

   _____

34. What is a Rumel?

   _____

   _____

   _____

35. Discuss how a surgical technologist might maintain a "dry field" during peripheral vascular procedures.

_____

_____

_____

36. Once your patient has been systemically heparinized, what should a surgical technologist have on her or his back table to prepare for this heparinized condition?

_____

_____

_____

37. What is the reversal agent for heparin sodium?

_____

_____

_____

38. What medication might be used to reduce vasospasm during a thrombectomy?

_____

_____

_____

39. During peripheral vascular procedures, the surgical technologist might have many different types of medication on the back table, including lidocaine, heparin, an antibiotic irrigation, a heparin irrigation, and Hypaque. What must a surgical technologist do to ensure the safe delivery of medication to the surgical patient?

_____

_____

_____

40. How does the contrast media used in angiography work?

_____

_____

_____

41. What is the difference between a vascular stent and a vascular graft?

_____

_____

_____

42. What is the difference between a thrombus and an embolus?

_____

_____

_____

43. Why are thrombi removed with an embolectomy catheter?

_____

_____

_____

44. Why would a patient need a renal access graft for hemodialysis?

_____

_____

_____

45. What is the difference between an A-V fistula and an A-V graft?

_____

_____

_____

46. What are pulmonary emboli? How are they prevented surgically?

_____

_____

_____

47. During carotid endarterectomy, it may be necessary to temporarily occlude the carotid arteries while plaque is removed. What is the system for removing the vascular clamps at the end of the procedure?

_____

_____

_____

48. Is saphenous vein harvesting a graft in situ? Why or why not?

_____

_____

_____

49. Describe the differences between the following bypass procedures.

   A. Axillofemoral bypass:

   _____

   _____

   B. Femoral popliteal bypass:

   _____

   _____

   C. Saphenous femoropopliteal bypass:

   _____

   _____

   D. Femorofemoral bypass:

   _____

   _____

Internet Exercises

1. Do an Internet search on peripheral vascular disease. In particular, go to the website for the Texas Heart Institute (THI). You will be searching the site for the following areas of interest:

   A. Where is the THI located? Who is the THI's major sponsor? Are there other hospitals in the area?

   _____

   _____

   _____

   B. Who is Dr. Denton Cooley? Why is his career significant to a surgical technologist?

   _____

   _____

   _____

   C. How is Dr. Denton Cooley associated with the institute?

   _____

   _____

   _____

   D. Which types of patient education are offered through the Texas Heart Institute? Do other sites offer this type of education for patients with peripheral vascular disease? What are they? Which types of education do they offer patients and staff members?

   _____

   _____

   _____

   E. List the Internet sites used. _____

   _____

2. Do an Internet search on PAD (peripheral artery disease). Look for sites that will answer the following questions:

   A. Which sites that you found provided the most information?

   _____

   _____

   _____

   _____

B. Which sites were written for the general public?

_____

_____

_____

C. Which sites were written for allied health professionals?

_____

_____

_____

D. What did you learn about the effects of smoking on the peripheral vascular system?

_____

_____

_____

E. Which peripheral vascular diseases are directly linked to smoking?

_____

_____

_____

F. Does the patient's risk for these diseases decrease if she or he stops smoking after a 40-year habit?

_____

_____

_____

G. List the Internet sites used.

_____

_____

Chapter 29
Cardiothoracic Surgery

Key Terms

Write the definition for each term.

1. Aneurysm: _____

   _____

2. Arrhythmia: _____

   _____

3. Asystole: _____

   _____

4. Bolster: _____

   _____

5. Bucking: _____

   _____

6. Cardioplegia: _____

   _____

7. Coarctation: _____

   _____

8. Commissurotomy: _____

   _____

9. Congenital: _____

   _____

273

10. Cross-clamp: _____

_____

11. Dysrhythmia: _____

_____

12. Fibrillation: _____

_____

13. Fusiform aneurysm: _____

_____

14. Infarction: _____

_____

15. Ischemia: _____

_____

16. Lobectomy: _____

_____

17. Mediastinum: _____

_____

18. Off-pump procedure: _____

_____

19. Pacemaker: _____

_____

20. Pneumonectomy: _____

_____

21. Pre-clotting: _____

_____

22. Regurgitant valve: _____

_____

23. Saccular aneurysm: _____

_____

24. Shunt: _____

_____

25. Stenosis: _____

_____

26. Sternotomy: _____

_____

27. Syncope: _____

_____

28. Tag: _____

_____

29. Tamponade: _____

_____

30. Vasoconstriction: _____

_____

31. Wedge resection: _____

_____

Labeling

32. Label the illustration using the following terms:

left atrium	right ventricle	papillary muscle	openings to coronary arteries
right atrium	interventricular septum	tricuspid valve	pulmonary vein
superior vena cava	mitral valve	aorta	chordae tendineae
left ventricle	pulmonary trunk		

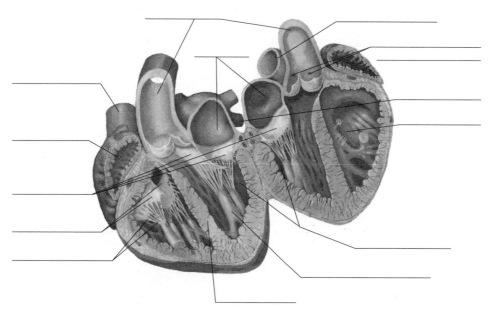

33. Label the illustration using the following terms:

rib	pulmonary vein	visceral pleura	pulmonary trunk
left lung	pulmonary artery	right lung	primary bronchus
esophagus	heart	vertebra	intrapleural space
sternum	parietal pleura	aorta	

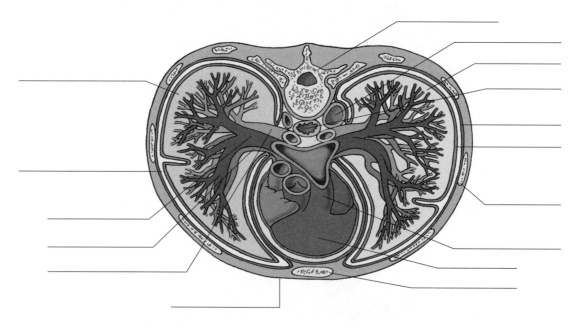

Short Answers

34. The conduction system of the heart causes the heart to beat. Explain how that occurs.

_____

_____

_____

35. Why would your surgeon want a vascular graft?

_____

_____

_____

36. What is the difference between the two different types of vascular grafts?

_____

_____

_____

37. How would a surgical technologist make a Rumel tourniquet? Why would the surgeon need one?

_____

_____

_____

38. Describe three diagnostic cardiothoracic procedures listed below.

    A. bronchoscopy:

    _____

    _____

    _____

    B. mediastinoscopy:

    _____

    _____

    _____

C. scalene node biopsy:

_____

_____

_____

39. Discuss the care of surgical specimens during an endoscopic procedure.

_____

_____

_____

40. What is the difference between open procedures done on the heart and open heart procedures? Give an example of each type.

_____

_____

_____

41. Name the five drugs that might be used in cardiothoracic procedures and their uses.

A. _____

B. _____

C. _____

D. _____

E. _____

42. What is a thoracostomy?

_____

_____

_____

Internet Exercises

1. Do an Internet search of heart transplants and be prepared to discuss in class the answers to the following questions:

   A. Where is the closest organ transplant hospital in your area? See if you can locate it on the Internet. List its site.

   _____

   _____

   _____

   B. Search the Internet for patients who have received a heart transplant.

   _____

   _____

   _____

   C. How many of the sites found were from parents who have created sites for their children?

   _____

   _____

   _____

   D. How many of the sites found were from families of donors?

   _____

   _____

   _____

   E. How has this increased your awareness of organ donation?

   _____

   _____

   _____

   F. How do you think this information will impact your future regarding organ donation?

   _____

   _____

   _____

2. Do an Internet search on the LAVD (left assistive ventricular device) and also on Dr. Michael DeBakey, a doctor involved in designing and researching the device, then answer the following questions:

A. Who is Dr. Michael DeBakey?

_____

_____

_____

B. Why should we trust his research on the LAVD?

_____

_____

_____

C. The LAVD is primarily being used to "bridge" patients to a heart transplant. What does that mean?

_____

_____

_____

D. What did your Internet search reveal about the future of the LAVD?

_____

_____

_____

Chapter 30
Pediatric Surgery

Key Terms

Write the definition for each term.

1. Aganglionic: _____

_____

2. Atresia: _____

_____

3. Branchial cleft cyst: _____

_____

4. Choanal: _____

_____

5. Endocardial cushion: _____

_____

6. Exstrophy: _____

_____

7. Gastroschisis: _____

_____

8. Nephroblastoma: _____

_____

9. Omphalocele: _____

_____

10. Sternocleidomastoid: _____

    _____

11. Thermogenesis: _____

    _____

12. Thyroglossal duct: _____

    _____

Short Answers

Fill in the age groups for the following pediatric patients:

13. A. Neonate: _____

    B. Infant: _____

    C. Toddler: _____

    D. Preschooler: _____

    E. School-age child: _____

    F. Adolescent: _____

14. Discuss the following specific problems regarding the physiological needs of pediatric patients in the following areas:

    A. Airway and pulmonary management:

    _____

    _____

    _____

    B. Cardiovascular:

    _____

    _____

    _____

C. Temperature regulation:

_____

_____

_____

D. Metabolism:

_____

_____

_____

E. Fluid and electrolyte balance:

_____

_____

_____

15. Discuss the common fears and psychological needs of children in the surgical suite.

_____

_____

_____

16. What special considerations will be given to pediatric instrumentation?

_____

_____

_____

Matching

Match each term with the correct definition.

A. choanal atresia

B. branchial cleft cyst

C. gastroschisis

D. omphalocele

E. anorectoplasty

F. reduction of volvulus

G. imperforate anus

_____ 17. A congenital malformation in which variable amounts of abdominal contents protrude into the base of the umbilical cord

_____ 18. Obstruction at the anorectal level resulting from congenital atresia

_____ 19. An embryonic developmental defect that develops from the primitive branchial apparatus

_____ 20. The absence of a normal anal opening

_____ 21. A congenital anomaly of the anterior skull base characterized by closure of one or both posterior nasal cavities

_____ 22. An abdominal wall defect caused by the failure of the abdominal wall to develop just to the right of the umbilical ring

_____ 23. The clockwise rotation or twisting of a loop of intestine around itself, affecting its own blood supply

Short Answers

24. Discuss the four classes of imperforate anus.

_____

_____

_____

_____

25. *Place an X next to all of the congenital birth defects*

_____ intussusception

_____ volvulus

_____ Wilms' tumor

_____ bladder exstrophy

_____ Hirschsprung's disease

26. Explain the three stages of reconstruction of a bladder exstrophy.

    A. 1st Stage:

    _____

    _____

    B. 2nd Stage:

    _____

    _____

    C. 3rd Stage:

    _____

    _____

27. Explain the difference between each of the three types of approaches to choanal atresia repair.

    A. _____

    _____

    _____

    B. _____

    _____

    _____

    C. _____

    _____

    _____

    _____

28. Branchial cleft cysts, sinuses, and fistulas are classified into first, second, third, and fourth branchial abnormalities. Differentiate between the four types.

    A. _____

    _____

    _____

B. _____

_____

_____

C. _____

_____

_____

D. _____

_____

_____

29. What is Hirschsprung's disease?

_____

_____

_____

Internet Exercises

1. Go online and research the difference between an omphalocele, which is a congenital malformation, and a common umbilical hernia. After your Internet search, answer the following questions:

A. Which websites were helpful when researching the two procedures and anomalies?

_____

_____

_____

B. Which websites were *not* helpful in your search?

_____

_____

_____

C. What are the *major* differences between the two procedures?

_____

_____

_____

D. How are the procedures alike?

_____

_____

_____

E. Did any of the websites you used to research these two subjects offer information on a related condition called "gastroschisis?"

_____

_____

_____

F. Did any of the websites you used to research this assignment offer links to other pediatric anomalies?

_____

_____

_____

2. Go online to search for several specific pediatric birth defects. Once you find a site where you can research several defects at once, answer the following questions:

A. How many of the pediatric operations occur as a single anomaly?

_____

_____

_____

B. How many occur with premature infants?

_____

_____

_____

C. How many occur with premature infants born as quadruplets or sextuplets, etc.?

_____

_____

_____

Be prepared for your next class lecture with your research findings and a list of the websites used. Your instructor may conduct a classroom discussion based on your research.

Chapter 31
Neurosurgery

Key Terms

Write the definition for each term.

1. Acoustic neuroma: _____

   _____

2. A-V malformation: _____

   _____

3. Berry aneurysm: _____

   _____

4. Bur: _____

   _____

5. Central nervous system: _____

   _____

6. Cerebral aqueduct: _____

   _____

7. Cerebral peduncle: _____

   _____

8. Cerebrospinal fluid: _____

   _____

9. Corpora quadrigemina: _____

   _____

10. Cryosurgery: _____

_____

11. Endoneurium: _____

_____

12. Epineurium: _____

_____

13. Fascicles: _____

_____

14. Foramen magnum: _____

_____

15. Galea: _____

_____

16. Gray commissure: _____

_____

17. Gray matter: _____

_____

18. Hypothermia: _____

_____

19. Interventricular foramen: _____

_____

20. In vitro: _____

_____

21. Ligamentum flavum: _____

_____

22. Meninges: _____

_____

23. Pericranium: _____

_____

24. Perineurium: _____

_____

25. Rami: _____

_____

26. Scalp: _____

_____

27. Skull: _____

_____

28. Stereotactic: _____

_____

29. Suture: _____

_____

30. Trephination: _____

_____

31. Trephine: _____

_____

32. Ventricle: _____

_____

33. Vertebra: _____

_____

34. Vertebral lamina: _____

_____

35. White matter: _____

_____

Labeling

36. Label the drawing of the meninges using the following terms:

Arachnoid granulation   Choroid plexus of third ventricle   Interventricular foramen
Cerebral aqueduct   Dura mater   Subarachnoid space
Choroid plexus of fourth ventricle   Foramen in fourth ventricle   Superior sagittal sinus
Choroid plexus of lateral ventricle

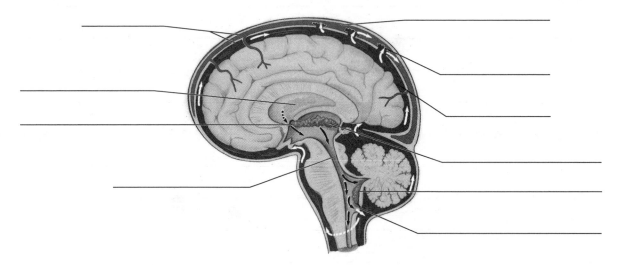

37. Label the two drawings of the brain using the following terms:

midbrain	temporal lobe	gustatory area
cerebellum	occipital lobe	wernicke's area
pons	Broca's area	lateral sulcus
medulla	longitudinal fissure	pituitary gland
gyrus	precentral gyrus somatomotor cortex	thalamus
sulcus	central sulcus	hypothalamus
frontal lobe	postcentral gyrus somatosensory cortex	spinal cord
parietal lobe	gnostic area	

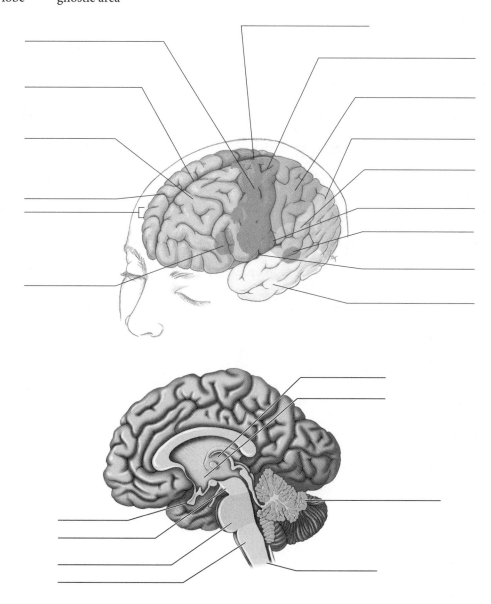

Short Answers

38. What is the difference between the two divisions of the central nervous system?

_____

_____

_____

39. Name the 12 pairs of cranial nerves.

A. _____

_____

B. _____

_____

C. _____

_____

D. _____

_____

E. _____

_____

F. _____

_____

G. _____

_____

H. _____

_____

I. _____

_____

J. _____

_____

K. _____

_____

L. _____

_____

40. How many spinal nerves are there, and how are they arranged?

_____

_____

_____

41. What is a Mayfield table, and when is it used?

_____

_____

42. What special considerations might be utilized in prepping and draping a neurological patient who is undergoing a craniotomy?

_____

_____

43. Research the suction tips used in neurosurgery, and list the specifics involved in the instrumentation.

_____

_____

44. Describe the uses of the Frazier suction tip in neurosurgery.

_____

_____

45. The use of irrigation solution during neurosurgery is quite different from other types of operations. Research the use of irrigation solutions in neurosurgery and list the solutions.

_____

_____

46. Describe the difference between angiography and myelography.

_____

_____

47. Name the two different types of peripheral nerve repair.

_____

_____

48. Why would your patient need a sympathectomy?

_____

_____

49. What are the four common indications for a laminectomy?

A. _____

_____

B. _____

_____

C. _____

_____

D. _____

_____

50. During a laminectomy there will be three separate specimens. Name them.

A. _____

_____

B. _____

_____

C. _____

_____

51. What is the surgical technologist's role in caring for the specimen during a laminectomy?

_____

_____

52. Why is a biploar ESU preferred during a craniotomy?

_____

_____

53. Describe the major components in the spinal fixation system. There are many types and manufacturers, but they all have the same major components.

_____

_____

54. Why is a craniotomy performed?

_____

_____

55. What is the difference in procedure between a patient who is diagnosed with an epidural hematoma and a patient who is diagnosed with a subdural hematoma?

_____

_____

56. Why is a craniectomy performed? Describe the typical patient for this procedure.

_____

_____

57. Why would someone need decompression of a cranial nerve?

_____

_____

58. What is a myelomeningocele, and how is it corrected?

_____

_____

Internet Exercises

1. Go online to the National Geographic website, and find an archived article entitled "Quiet Miracles of the Brain" from June 1995. The article contains marvelous color anatomical and functional pictures of the brain that will help you study for this chapter. Additionally, the author describes and discusses in depth several case studies about brain dysfunctions and disorders. Read the article (it is about 40 pages long, so allow adequate time for the assignment), and keep in mind the following questions:

   A. What did you learn about the function of the brain that you did not already know? _____

   _____

   B. What did you learn about a diagnostic procedure that you did not already know? _____

   _____

   C. How did you feel about the specific patients described in the case studies?

      1. the twins with schizophrenia? _____

      _____

      2. the older woman with Alzheimer's disease? _____

      _____

      3. the middle-age woman with amnesia? _____

      _____

Take notes if necessary, and come to class prepared to answer the questions during a classroom forum.

2. Do an Internet search for "medical mnemonics." (You did this exercise for the Orthopedics unit.) Find a web page that will allow you to look up ways to remember the 12 cranial nerves, neurological anatomy, pathology, and diseases.

   Memorize several of the mnemonics that might help you in this unit. List the study tools that you thought were most helpful as well as the website. You may be asked to share these tools with your classmates in an open classroom discussion. Have fun!

   _____

   _____

   _____

   _____

   _____